High-Yield Pathology

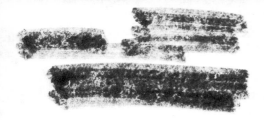

High-Yield Pathology

Ivan Damjanov, M.D., Ph.D.

Professor of Pathology

The University of Kansas School of Medicine

Kansas City, Kansas

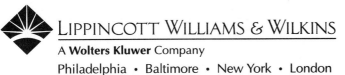

LIPPINCOTT WILLIAMS & WILKINS

A **Wolters Kluwer** Company

Philadelphia · Baltimore · New York · London
Buenos Aires · Hong Kong · Sydney · Tokyo

Editor: Elizabeth Nieginski
Editorial Director: Julie P. Scardiglia
Development Editor: Melanie Cann
Managing Editor: Marette Magargle-Smith
Marketing Manager: Kelley Ray

351 West Camden Street
Baltimore, Maryland 21201-2436 USA

530 Walnut Street
Philadelphia, Pennsylvania 19106 USA

The publisher is not responsible (as a matter of product liability, negligence, or otherwise) for any injury resulting from any material contained herein. This publication contains information relating to general principles of medical care which should not be construed as specific instructions for individual patients. Manufacturers' product information and package inserts should be reviewed for current information, including contraindications, dosages, and precautions.

Printed in the United States of America

Library of Congress Cataloging-in-Publication Data

Damjanov, Ivan.
    High-yield pathology/Ivan Damjanov.
        p.; cm.—(High-yield)
    Includes index.
    ISBN 0–7817–2367–1
    1. Pathology—Outlines, syllabi, etc. 2. Pathology—Examinations, questions, etc. I.
Title. II. High-yield series.
    [DNLM: 1. Pathology—Examination Questions. 2. Pathology—Outlines. QY 18.2
D161h 2000]
    RB120.D348 2000
    616.07'076—dc21
                                                               00-032737

The publishers have made every effort to trace the copyright holders for borrowed material. If they have inadvertently overlooked any, they will be pleased to make the necessary arrangements at the first opportunity.

To purchase additional copies of this book call our customer service department at **(800) 638-3030** or fax orders to **(301) 824–7390.** International customers should call **(301) 714-2324.**

00 01 02

1 2 3 4 5 6 7 8 9 10

Contents

Preface

The review books that comprise the *High-Yield* series have been popular with medical students all over the United States. I spend quite a bit of time in the company of medical students, and it was from them initially that I learned that a concise review of sophomore pathology would be a welcome addition to this very successful series. My friends in our university bookstore echoed the students' point of view and encouraged me to undertake the task of writing such a book. The publisher was equally enthusiastic and, in due time, with the assistance of an experienced editor, *High-Yield Pathology* became a reality.

High-Yield Pathology covers what I think every medical student should know after completing the sophomore pathology course. It also reflects my belief that understanding a selected body of facts well is more important than possessing superficial knowledge of many facts of varying significance. Readers will notice that I have an intolerance for trivia, and I do not encourage rote memorization (although occasionally, I will resort to mnemonics or other tricks that enable the reader to place bare facts into a context that allows for easier retention of the information). There is a significant difference between *knowing* something and *knowing about* something.

Like all other books in this series, *High-Yield Pathology* was written in an outline format designed for quick review. From my discussions with students, I foresee that some will use it just for that—a brief review before the final course examination and the United States Medical Licensing Examination (USMLE) Step 1. These students follow the educational philosophy that textbooks should be used for acquiring the knowledge during the course, whereas concise review books are most appropriate as adjuncts to exam preparation. Students belonging to the opposite camp will buy the book at the beginning of their pathology course and use it as a study guide (i.e., a "navigational tool" for sailing through the prescribed textbook and lecture notes). The students of this persuasion believe, and not without foundation, that whatever information is emphasized in two books (i.e., the textbook and the review book) must be important and is truly "high yield." My hopes are that both groups will find the present book useful and compatible with their own style of studying. I wish you all good luck!

Ivan Damjanov, M.D., Ph.D.
Kansas City, Kansas

1

Cell Injury

I. INTRODUCTION. Cells are in homeostasis with the extracellular fluid and respond to changes in their environment.

   A. Adaptation is the cell's response to prolonged stress.

   B. Cell injury. If the cell's ability to adapt is overtaxed, cellular injury results. Initially, cellular injury may be **reversible** (referred to as **hydropic change),** but in the face of prolonged or severe stress, the damage becomes **irreversible** (referred to as **necrosis).**

   C. Cell death. There are two forms of cell death—**necrosis,** the ultimate result of irreversible cell injury, and **apoptosis** (programmed cell death).

II. CELL INJURY

   A. Causes of cell injury include:

   1. Oxygen deficiency

   2. **Free radicals,** especially oxygen radicals [e.g., superoxide ($O_2\cdot$), hydrogen peroxide (H_2O_2), and hydroxyl radical ($OH\cdot$)]

   3. **Chemical** or **physical agents**

   4. **Biological agents** (e.g., cytokines, oncogenes)

   B. Ultrastructural signs of cell injury (Figure 1-1)

   1. Seen in both reversible and irreversible cell injury
      a. **Cellular swelling.** Diminished activity of the sodium pump in the cell membrane causes an influx of sodium (leading to an isosmotic gain of water, and swelling of the cell) and an efflux of potassium.
      b. **Mitochondrial swelling** results in reduced aerobic respiration.
      c. **Dilatation and degranulation of the rough endoplasmic reticulum** results in cessation of protein synthesis.
      d. **Autophagocytosis** is the ingestion of damaged organelles by lysosomes.

   2. Seen only in **irreversible cell injury**
      a. **Cell membrane rupture** shrinking nucleus
      b. **Nuclear changes,** including **pyknosis** (nuclear condensation), **karyolysis** (loss of nuclear chromatin), and **karyorrhexis** (nuclear fragmentation)

1

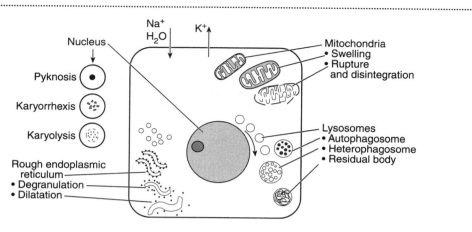

Figure 1-1. Ultrastructural signs of cell injury. Changes are seen in the mitochondria, lysosomes, rough endoplasmic reticulum, and nucleus. Nuclear changes denote irreversible cell injury. H_2O = water; K^+ = potassium; Na^+ = sodium.

III. CELL DEATH

A. **Necrosis** is a morphologic sign of cell death in a living tissue. Several forms of necrosis are recognized (Figure 1-2).

1. **Coagulative necrosis,** typically caused by ischemia (infarct), is the most common form of necrosis. The necrotic tissue appears pale and firm and retains its normal shape because no enzymatic lysis occurs—enzymes, like all other proteins, have been "coagulated" (i.e., inactivated).

2. **Liquefactive necrosis** is typically found in the brain or in an abscess (i.e., a pus-filled cavity). Tissue is softened ("liquefied") through the action of enzymes released from brain cells or, in the case of an abscess, polymorphonuclear neutrophils (PMNs).

3. **Caseous necrosis** is typically seen in tuberculosis and certain fungal granulomas. The tissue appears cheesy; histologically, it consists of granular material surrounded by epithelioid and multinucleated giant cells.

4. **Fat necrosis** may be caused by trauma to adipose cells, or induced by lipolytic enzymes released during disease states (e.g., lipase release in acute pancreatitis). Free fatty acids released from fat cells bind with calcium to form white specks composed of calcium soaps.

5. **Fibrinoid necrosis** is typically seen in arteries, arterioles, or glomerular capillaries damaged by autoimmune diseases. Blood vessels are impregnated by fibrin and other serum proteins and appear magenta-red in histologic sections.

"Wet gangrene" is a clinical term for ischemic necrosis accompanied by bacterial decomposition, which leads to partial liquefaction of the tissues. "Dry gangrene" ("mummification") refers to noninfected ischemic necrosis accompanied by drying of the tissues.

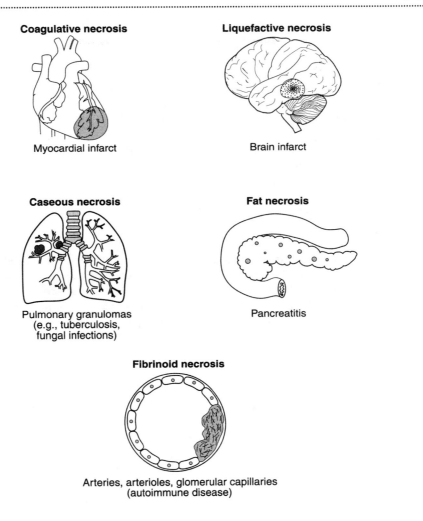

Figure 1-2. Forms of necrosis.

B. **Apoptosis** is based on activation of specific "death pathway genes." Apoptosis may be physiologic or pathologic.

   1. Examples of physiologic apoptosis include the:

      a. Programmed death of embryonic cells in the limb buds (leading to the formation of fingers and toes)

      b. Predetermined death of cells on the surface of the intestinal mucosa

      c. Hormone-induced cell death of endometrial cells at the end of the menstrual cycle

   2. Examples of pathologic apoptosis include:

      a. Hepatitis virus-induced liver cell apoptosis ("acidophilic bodies")

    b. Immune injury-related skin keratinocytes ("Civatte bodies")

    c. Corticosteroid-induced atrophy of the neonatal thymus

IV. ADAPTATION (Figure 1-3)

A. Atrophy is a reduction in the size of an organ or tissue owing to either cell loss or a reduction in the size of cells. Typical examples are atrophy of the brain in Alzheimer disease or thinning of the bones in osteoporosis.

B. Hypertrophy is an increase in the size of an organ or tissue owing to enlargement of constituent cells. Typical examples include the response of the heart and skeletal muscles to prolonged effort.

C. Hyperplasia is an increase in the size of an organ owing to an increased number of cells. Hyperplasia can be induced by hormones (e.g., endometrial hyperplasia induced by estrogen) or viruses (e.g., common wart, caused by human papillomavirus).

> **In many instances, hypertrophy and hyperplasia occur coincidentally (e.g., benign prostatic hyperplasia, hypertrophy of the urinary bladder secondary to urethral obstruction). In clinical practice, such changes are designated as either hypertrophy or hyperplasia; these designations reflect time-honored conventions!**

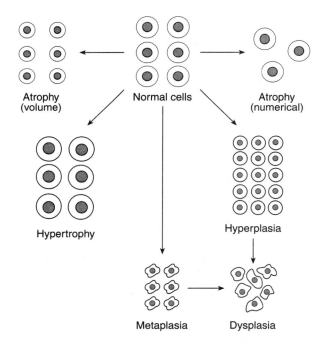

Figure 1-3. Adaptations of the cell caused by chronic stress or injury include atrophy, hypertrophy, hyperplasia, metaplasia, and dysplasia.

D. **Metaplasia** is the transformation of one tissue cell type into another. Examples include squamous metaplasia of the bronchial epithelium as a result of cigarette smoking, and metaplasia of the squamous epithelium of the esophagus into intestinal or gastric epithelium owing to reflux of gastric juice (Barrett esophagus).

E. **Dysplasia** (i.e., atypical hyperplasia or metaplasia) is a premalignant transformation of normal epithelia. Typically, dysplasia is found in the cervix, where it may progress to carcinoma *in situ* and invasive carcinoma.

V. ACCUMULATIONS AND DEPOSITS. Chronic cell injury or metabolic disorders can lead to the accumulation of substances in cells and the extracellular matrix.

A. Intracellular accumulations

1. **Glycogen** accumulates in the liver, muscles, or kidneys in patients with inborn errors of glycogen metabolism or diabetes mellitus.

2. **Fat** accumulates in the liver in obese patients and patients with chronic alcoholism.

3. **Protein** accumulates in the proximal renal tubules in patients with proteinuria.

4. **Pigments** that accumulate in various cells include **lipofuscin** (i.e., the brown pigment formed in the lysosomes of elderly people), **melanin** (i.e., the brown pigment typically found in melanocytes and melanomas), and **hemosiderin** (i.e., the iron-rich brown pigment derived from hemolyzed red blood cells).

> **NB**
>
> **Hemochromatosis is a genetic disorder of iron absorption characterized by the deposition of hemosiderin in the spleen, liver, and bone marrow. Patients present with cirrhosis, diabetes, and skin discoloration ("bronzed diabetes").**

B. **Calcification.** Deposits of calcium salts in the cells and extracellular matrix can be classified as dystrophic or metastatic.

1. **Dystrophic calcification** involves damaged or dead tissue (e.g., calcification of atherosclerotic blood vessels and scarred aortic valves).

2. **Metastatic calcification** is secondary to hypercalcemia and is typically associated with hyperparathyroidism, hypervitaminosis D, or end-stage renal disease. Metastatic calcification is most often seen in the kidneys, lungs, or stomach.

C. **Amyloid deposition.** The deposition of amyloid, a proteinaceous substance, between the cells of various tissues leads to a group of clinical conditions collectively known as "amyloidosis."

1. **Histologic appearance of amyloid.** Amyloid is extracellular fibrillar material formed from a variety of polypeptides.
  a. By light microscopy, amyloid appears like hyalin (homogeneous eosinophilic material).
  b. Although biochemically heterogeneous, all forms of amyloid have the following common features:
    (1) β-Pleated sheet structure on x-ray crystallography and infrared spectroscopy
    (2) Beaded fibrillar appearance on electron microscopy

(3) Apple-green birefringence when stained with Congo red dye and examined under polarized light

2. Important clinical forms of amyloidosis

a. Primary amyloidosis, a typical feature of multiple myeloma, is characterized by deposits of AL amyloid, which is derived from the immunoglobulin light chain. AL amyloid deposits are found in the kidneys, blood vessels, and heart.

b. Secondary amyloidosis is characterized by deposits of AA amyloid, which is derived from serum amyloid-associated protein. Serum amyloid-associated protein is produced by the liver in chronic suppurative or autoimmune diseases, and in neoplastic diseases (e.g., renal cancer). AA amyloid deposits are found in the kidneys, liver, and spleen.

c. Familial amyloidosis results from deposits of abnormal transthyretin in the nerves.

d. Localized amyloid deposits are typical of Alzheimer disease (deposits are seen in the cerebral cortex) and medullary carcinoma of the thyroid.

2

Inflammation and Repair

I. INTRODUCTION. Inflammation is the body's reaction to injury. The purpose of this reaction is twofold—it eliminates the cause of the injury, and then initiates the repair and healing of injured tissue.

   A. Causes of inflammation include infections, immune reactions, foreign bodies, necrotic tissue, and tumors.

   B. Types of inflammation. Inflammation may be acute or chronic.

   1. Acute inflammation is usually the result of infection or tissue necrosis (e.g., infarct).

   2. Chronic inflammation. Causes include:
   a. Nonhealing acute processes (e.g., chronic abscess or ulcer)
   b. Bacteria and other infectious agents that cannot be eliminated (e.g., *Mycobacterium tuberculosis* in tuberculosis, HIV in AIDS)
   c. Foreign bodies or inorganic material
   d. Immune reactions, which tend to be autocatalytic

II. ACUTE INFLAMMATION. The classic signs of acute inflammation are **rubor** (redness), **tumor** (swelling), **calor** (heat), **dolor** (pain), and **functio laesa** (impaired function). The vascular and cellular events that characterize acute inflammation are responsible for these clinical signs.

   A. The inflammatory response

   1. Vascular events. Following transient arteriolar constriction, the arterioles dilate, allowing an influx of blood under increased pressure **(active hyperemia).**
   a. The increased intravascular pressure, combined with increased vessel wall permeability, leads to transudation of fluid into the perivascular spaces **(edema).**
   b. Dilatation of flooded venules contributes to **stasis of blood in the capillaries** by slowing outflow.

   2. Cellular events. Polymorphonuclear neutrophils **(PMNs)** are the primary effector cells in acute inflammation. Figure 2-1 illustrates the sequence of events that occurs in response to a bacterial infection:
   a. Margination. The PMNs, which usually travel toward the center of the vessel, settle toward the sides of the vessel as blood flow through the vessel slows.
   b. Activation. Mediators of inflammation trigger the appearance of molecules known as **selectins** and **integrins** on the surfaces of endothelial cells and PMNs, respectively.

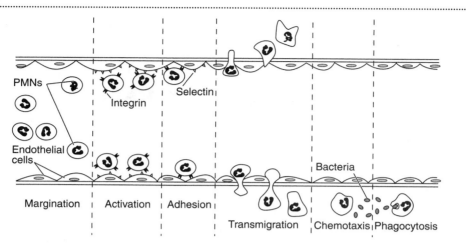

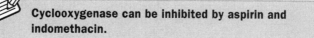

Figure 2-1. Sequence of events in the polymorphonuclear neutrophil (PMN) response to bacterial infection.

    c. Adhesion of the PMNs to endothelial cells is mediated by selectins and integrins.

    d. Transmigration (diapedesis). The PMNs cross the vessel wall, moving into the interstitial space.

    e. Chemotaxis. The PMNs move toward the site of infection, in response to chemotactic factors released by bacteria or formed from activated complement, chemokines, or arachidonic acid derivatives.

    f. Phagocytosis. The PMNs ingest the bacteria and kill them.

B. Chemical mediators account for the vascular and cellular events that occur during the acute inflammatory response.

    1. Cell-derived mediators include histamine, arachidonic acid derivatives, nitric oxide (NO), and cytokines.

        a. Histamine, which causes arteriolar and venular dilation and increased vascular permeability, is released from circulating basophils, tissue mast cells, and platelets.

        b. Arachidonic acid is metabolized through two pathways.

            (1) The **cyclooxygenase pathway** leads to the synthesis of:

                (a) Prostaglandins (PGD_2, PGE_2, PGF_2), which cause vasodilatation

                (b) Prostacyclin (PGI_2), which causes vasodilatation and inhibits platelet aggregation

                (c) Thromboxane A_2, which causes vasoconstriction and promotes platelet aggregation

> **NB**
>
> **Cyclooxygenase can be inhibited by aspirin and indomethacin.**

            (2) The **lipoxygenase pathway** leads to the synthesis of:

                (a) Leukotriene B_4, which is chemotactic

(b) Leukotrienes C_4, D_4, and E_4, which cause vasoconstriction, bronchospasm, and increased vascular permeability

c. **NO** is a short-lived reactant. When released from endothelial cells, NO causes relaxation of the vascular smooth muscle cells, leading to dilatation of the vessels. When released from macrophages, NO is microbicidal and cytotoxic.

d. **Cytokines** are polypeptides and include the **interleukins** (e.g., IL-1, IL-2) and **tumor necrosis factor (TNF).** Cytokines are primarily released from macrophages and lymphocytes, but can be released from many other cells as well.

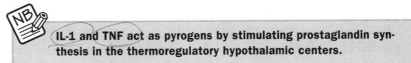

IL-1 and TNF act as pyrogens by stimulating prostaglandin synthesis in the thermoregulatory hypothalamic centers.

2. **Plasma-derived mediators** include **kinins** (e.g., bradykinin), **coagulation proteins** (e.g., fibrin, fibrin split product), **fibrinolytic proteins** (e.g., plasmin), and **complement.** These mediators are typically activated by factor XII (Hageman factor; Figure 2-2).

C. **Pathologic types** of acute inflammation. The pathologic type depends on the type of exudate and the extent of tissue destruction (Table 2-1).

III. CHRONIC INFLAMMATION.
Prolonged inflammation is mediated by cells that have a longer lifespan than PMNs and usually involves tissue destruction and repair.

A. The inflammatory response

1. **Vascular events** are similar to those that take place in acute inflammation, but include **angiogenesis** as well.

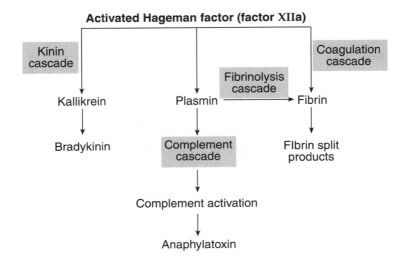

Figure 2-2. Activation of Hageman factor (factor XIIa) induces the kinin, complement, coagulation, and fibrinolysis cascades, resulting in the creation of the plasma-derived mediators of inflammation (i.e., kinins, coagulation proteins, and complement).

Table 2-1
Types of Inflammation

Type of Inflammation	Exudate	Clinical Examples
Serous	Serum-like clear fluid containing few cells	Herpes labialis, tuberculous pleural effusion
Fibrinous	Contains fibrin (polymerized fibrinogen)	Fibrinous pericarditis of rheumatic fever
Fibrinopurulent	Contains fibrin and PMNs	Streptococcal pharyngitis
Purulent	Contains PMNs, which turn into pus as they decompose	Staphylococcal furuncles ("boils"), abscess, empyema
Pseudomembranous	"Pseudomembrane" formed from necrosis of the superficial layer of mucosa and composed of fibrin, mucus, PMNs, and cell debris	Diphtherial pharyngitis, pseudo-membranous colitis (*Clostridium difficile* infection)
Ulcerative	Cell debris, PMNs, or granulation tissue	Syphilis chancre, peptic ulcer, ulcerative colitis

PMNs = polymorphonuclear neutrophils.

   2. Cellular events. Chronic inflammation is mediated by **macrophages, lymphocytes,** and **plasma cells. Eosinophils** participate in response to parasitic infections or allergic (immune-mediated) reactions.

B. Pathologic types of chronic inflammation. Histologically, chronic infection presents as:

   1. Interstitial diffuse infiltrates of lymphocytes, macrophages, and plasma cells (e.g., as seen in chronic pyelonephritis)

   2. Granulomas composed of epithelioid macrophages, multinucleated giant cells, and lymphocytes (e.g., as seen in sarcoidosis)

   3. Caseating granulomas (e.g., as seen in tuberculosis or fungal infection)

IV. REPAIR

A. Factors affecting healing. Healing of tissue injury or loss caused by inflammation depends on the type of cells that comprise the organ.

   1. Labile cells divide continuously; organs derived from these cells (e.g., the skin or intestinal mucosa) heal completely.

   2. Stable (facultative mitotic) cells are replaced by regeneration from remaining cells, which are stimulated to enter the mitotic cycle. Stable cells are found in the liver and kidney.

   3. Permanent (post-mitotic) cells, such as nerve cells and cardiac myocytes, cannot be replaced. Scar tissue is laid down in their stead.

B. Normal wound healing

   1. Healing by primary intention occurs in clean surgical wounds with apposed margins. It occurs in several phases:

   a. Blood fills the defect and coagulates, forming a **scab** (i.e., a meshwork composed of fibrin and fibronectin).

   b. Macrophages remove cell debris and secrete growth factors that stimulate angiogenesis and the ingrowth of fibroblasts and myofibroblasts, leading to the formation of **granulation tissue.**

   c. The epithelium regenerates, covering the surface defect.

   d. Deposition of an extracellular matrix, composed initially of collagen type III and later of collagen type I, occurs, resulting in **fibrous union.** By the end of the first week, 10% of the preoperative strength is regained and sutures can be removed safely.

   e. **Scar maturation** is a protracted phase during which cross-linking of collagen takes place. By the end of 3 months, 80% of the normal tensile strength of the tissue has been restored.

2. **Healing by secondary intention** occurs in large gaping or infected wounds. Typically, these wounds show:

   a. A more pronounced and prolonged inflammatory phase in which neutrophils may persist for days

   b. More abundant granulation tissue

   c. Wound contraction by myofibroblasts, which help to draw the margins of the wound closer to one another

C. **Abnormal wound healing**

1. **Delayed wound healing** may result from:

   a. Infection

   b. Mechanical factors (e.g., trauma, tension, foreign bodies)

   c. Malnutrition, poor circulation, or advanced age

   d. Drugs (e.g., corticosteroids, cytotoxic drugs)

2. **Wound dehiscence** (i.e., separation of the margins) may result from:

   a. Poor healing and weak scar formation

   b. Infection

   c. Mechanical factors that pull the edges of the wound apart (e.g., tension)

3. **Keloid formation.** Keloids are bulging, indurated masses resulting from abnormal excessive scar tissue formation. Keloid formation is more common in African-American patients.

3

Immunopathology

I. INTRODUCTION. The immune system provides a defense against substances perceived by the body as foreign ("non-self").

A. Types of immunity

1. Natural immunity does not require previous sensitization and is mediated by polymorphonuclear neutrophils (PMNs), macrophages, lymphocytes of the natural killer (NK) cell type, and protective substances (e.g., properdin, zymogen, complement).

2. Acquired immunity involves antibody production by B lymphocytes and delayed, cell-mediated immune reactions mounted by T lymphocytes.

B. Immune-mediated disorders may be systemic or localized to a particular organ. Major immune-mediated disorders include:

1. Hypersensitivity reactions

2. Autoimmune diseases

3. Immunodeficiency syndromes

4. Immunologic complications of organ transplantation

II. HYPERSENSITIVITY REACTIONS

A. Type I (anaphylactic) reactions (Figure 3-1)

1. Pathogenesis. Antigen reacts with IgE antibodies, which are bound to the surface of mast cells in tissue. The antigen-antibody reaction causes the mast cells to release granules rich in histamine and other vasoactive substances and stimulates the synthesis of arachidonic acid derivatives, platelet-activating factor (PAF), and cytokines, resulting in vasodilation and edema.

2. Clinical examples include **hay fever, bronchial asthma,** and **anaphylactic shock.**

B. Type II (antibody-mediated) reactions (Figure 3-2)

1. Complement-mediated lysis
   a. Pathogenesis. The binding of cytotoxic antibody to antigens expressed on a cell surface or basement membrane activates complement, which destroys or damages the antibody-coated structure.
   b. Clinical examples include **transfusion reactions, hemolytic disease of the newborn** (erythroblastosis fetalis), **autoimmune hemolytic anemia, Goodpasture syndrome,** and **pemphigus vulgaris.**

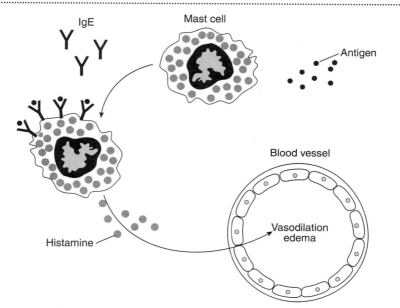

Figure 3-1.   Type I (anaphylactic) reaction. Antigen reacts with immunoglobulin E (*IgE*) antibodies on the surfaces of mast cells in tissue, causing the release of histamine and other vasoactive substances.

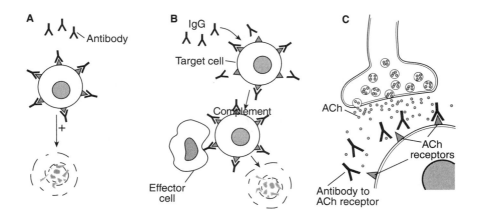

Figure 3-2.   Type II (antibody-mediated) reaction. (A) Complement-mediated lysis. The binding of cytotoxic antibody to antigens expressed on a cell surface activates complement, leading to lysis of the antibody-coated structure. (B) Antibody-dependent cell-mediated cytotoxicity (ADCC). Antigen on the surface of target cells binds with the Fab portion of immunoglobulin G (*IgG*), leaving the Fc portion exposed. The Fc portion then serves as a ligand for the receptors on various effector cells [e.g., natural killer (NK) cells, polymorphonuclear neutrophils (PMNs), or macrophages], which destroy the antibody-coated cells. (C) Antibody-mediated cell dysfunction. In myasthenia gravis, antibodies bind to the acetylcholine (*ACh*) receptors at the neuromuscular junction, displacing the physiologic stimulator (i.e., ACh) and resulting in periodic weakness.

2. Antibody-dependent cell-mediated cytotoxicity (ADCC)
   a. Pathogenesis. Antigen on the surface of target cells binds with the Fab portion of the antibody, leaving the Fc portion exposed. The Fc portion then serves as a ligand for the receptors on a variety of effector cells (e.g., NK cells, PMNs, macrophages, eosinophils).
   b. Clinical examples. ADCC reactions play a role in **autoimmune anemia, thrombocytopenia,** and **leukopenia.**

3. Antibody-mediated cell dysfunction
   a. Pathogenesis. Antibodies react with cell surface receptors for physiologic stimulators, leading to either the activation or inhibition of cell functions.
   b. Clinical examples include **myasthenia gravis,** a muscle disease characterized by periodic weakness owing to the binding of antibodies to acetylcholine (ACh) receptors at the neuromuscular junction, and **Graves disease,** a form of hyperthyroidism caused by the binding of antibodies to the thyroid-stimulating hormone (TSH) receptor on the surface of thyroid follicular cells.

C. Type III (immune complex-mediated) reactions (Figure 3-3)

   1. Pathogenesis. Antigen-antibody immune complexes circulate in the blood and are deposited along the basement membranes, typically on the glomerular basement membrane, on the synovial surface of joints, at the epidermal–dermal junction, and on serosal surfaces (e.g., pleurae). The deposited immune complexes activate complement, which amplifies the injury by attracting PMNs through chemotaxis.

   2. Clinical examples include **systemic lupus erythematosus (SLE), serum sickness, poststreptococcal glomerulonephritis, membranous nephropathy,** and **polyarteritis nodosa.**

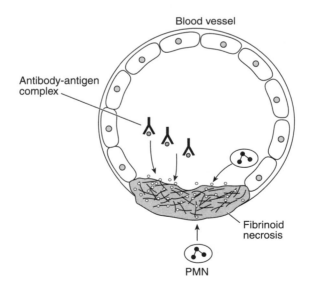

Figure 3-3. Type III (immune complex-mediated) reaction. The deposition of immune complexes leads to fibrinoid necrosis and the activation of complement. Complement compounds the injury by attracting polymorphonuclear neutrophils (*PMNs*) to the site, resulting in inflammation.

D. **Type IV (cell-mediated) reactions**

    1. **Delayed hypersensitivity reactions** are characterized by the formation of granulomas composed of **helper T (T_H) cells** and **macrophages** (Figure 3-4).

        a. **Pathogenesis**

            (1) Granuloma formation is initiated by T_H1 (CD4$^+$) cells. The T_H1 cells secrete cytokines, most notably interleukin-12 (IL-12) and interferon-γ (IFN-γ), which recruit macrophages to the site of injury.

            (2) The macrophages assume the appearance of epithelioid cells or fuse to form multinucleated giant cells. They secrete platelet-derived growth factor (PDGF) and tumor necrosis factor-β (TNF-β), substances that stimulate the ingrowth of fibroblasts (fibrosis).

        b. **Clinical examples** include **tuberculosis, leprosy,** and **deep fungal infections** (e.g., histoplasmosis, blastomycosis).

    2. **T cell-mediated cytotoxicity** is mediated by **CD8$^+$ cytotoxic T lymphocytes.**

        a. **Pathogenesis.** CD8$^+$ cytotoxic T lymphocytes kill the antigen-carrying cell directly.

        b. **Clinical examples** include **transplant rejection** and **contact dermatitis** ("poison ivy"). The response to some **viral infections** and **tumor immunity reactions** also involve CD8$^+$ cytotoxic lymphocytes.

III. AUTOIMMUNE DISEASES

A. General information

    1. The **etiology** and **pathogenesis** of the autoimmune diseases is unknown, but is most likely related to a loss of tolerance for "self" and a loss of suppressor T cell control over B cell functions, which leads to polyclonal B-cell activation.

        a. **Familial clustering** suggests a genetic basis.

        b. Some diseases (e.g., rheumatoid arthritis, Sjögren syndrome, ankylosing

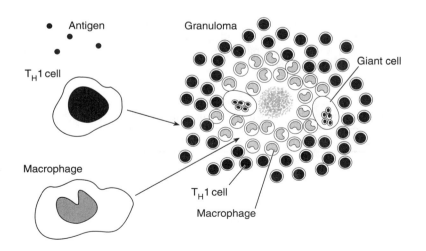

Figure 3-4. Delayed hypersensitivity reactions result in granuloma formation. Delayed hypersensitivity reactions are one form of type IV (cell-mediated) reaction; the other form is T cell-mediated cytotoxicity (not shown).

spondylitis) are **linked to specific human leukocyte antigen (HLA) haplotypes.**

2. Autoimmune disorders are **more common in women** than in men.

3. Autoimmune disorders may be **systemic** or **limited** to a specific organ or tissue.

B. Systemic lupus erythematosus (SLE), which typically affects young women, is characterized by the formation of autoantibodies to many endogenous antigens [e.g., DNA, RNA, nuclear proteins).

1. Clinical manifestations. Circulating immune complexes are deposited in many tissues, causing organ-specific lesions (Table 3-1).

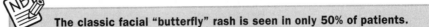

The classic facial "butterfly" rash is seen in only 50% of patients.

2. Diagnostic laboratory tests

a. An **antineutrophil antibody (ANA) test** is the best screening test for SLE. It is positive in 95% of patients with SLE, but it lacks specificity.

b. Antibody to double-stranded DNA (anti-dsDNA) is highly specific but is present in only 60% of patients with SLE.

c. Smith antibody to ribonucleoprotein (anti-Sm) is also highly specific for SLE, but only 30% of patients with SLE will have anti-Sm.

d. Serum complement levels. Depressed complement levels are a sign of disease activity.

e. Skin biopsy. A positive "lupus band test" is represented by granular deposits of immune complexes along the epidermal-dermal junction.

f. Renal biopsy is used to determine the type and severity of glomerular disease.

C. Progressive systemic sclerosis (PSS) is an autoimmune disease that predominantly affects women between the ages of 30 and 40 years. Widespread fibrosis results from the activation of T and B lymphocytes.

1. Forms

a. Diffuse disease. Pathologic findings include:

(1) Dermal sclerosis and epidermal atrophy (95% of patients)

(2) Gastrointestinal fibrosis, leading to motility disorders (especially in the esophagus)

Table 3-1
Organ-Specific Lesions in Systemic Lupus Erythematosus (SLE)

Organ or Tissue	Lesion	Incidence
Joints	Arthritis	95%
Skin	Dermatitis on sun-exposed areas	80%
Kidneys	Glomerulonephritis	60%
Serous surfaces	Pleuritis, pericarditis	50%
Blood	Hemolytic anemia, leukopenia, thrombocytopenia	50%
Heart	Libman-Sacks endocarditis	40%
Central nervous sytem (CNS) and eye	Microinfarcts	20%

(3) Musculoskeletal fibrosis, especially around the joints (leading to contractures)

(4) Interstitial fibrosis of the lungs

(5) Renal vascular fibrosis, leading to hypoperfusion and renal failure in 50% of affected patients

b. **Local disease** is usually limited to the distal extremities and face and is known as the **CREST variant** (**C**alcinosis, **R**aynaud's phenomenon, **E**sophageal motility dysfunction, **S**clerodactyly and **T**elangiectasia).

2. Diagnostic laboratory tests

a. **Antibodies to DNA topoisomerase I (Scl-70)** are present in 70% of patients with PSS.

b. **ANAs** are seen in 80% of patients with PSS.

c. **Anticentromere antibodies** are seen in 70% of patients with the CREST variant.

D. **Sjögren syndrome** is a disease primarily affecting middle-aged women.

1. **Primary sicca syndrome** affects the salivary and lacrimal glands and is manifested clinically by xerostomia (dry mouth) and xerophthalmia (dry eyes). Glands are enlarged and infiltrated with lymphocytes (predominantly CD4$^+$ cells). Sjögren syndrome antibodies (i.e., SS-A antibodies and SS-B antibodies) are seen in 90% of patients.

2. **Secondary sicca syndrome** is associated with other autoimmune diseases (e.g., rheumatoid arthritis, SLE, PSS, polymyositis). Salivary and lacrimal gland lesions are identical to those of primary sicca syndrome.

IV. IMMUNODEFICIENCY SYNDROMES

A. **Congenital immunodeficiency syndromes** result from impaired maturation of B or T lymphocytes. Patients present with recurrent infections.

1. **B-cell deficiencies** predispose to bacterial infections.

a. **Bruton agammaglobulinemia** is an X-linked failure of pre-B cells to differentiate into B cells and immunoglobulin-producing plasma cells. B cell areas of lymphoid tissues are atrophic and no plasma cells are present. Serum immunoglobulin levels are very low. Symptoms of reduced resistance to bacterial infections begin at approximately 6 months of age, after the stores of maternal antibodies have been depleted.

b. **Selective IgA deficiency** is the most common type of B-cell deficiency. Patients may be asymptomatic.

c. **Combined variable immunodeficiency** can affect both sexes and is characterized by a late onset, typically in the second or third decade. Hypogammaglobulinemia is characteristic.

2. **T-cell deficiencies** predispose to viral, fungal, protozoal, and intracellular bacterial infections. **DiGeorge syndrome** is a T-cell deficiency related to thymic aplasia associated with hypoparathyroidism.

3. **Combined B-cell and T-cell deficiency. Severe combined immunodeficiency (SCID)** includes several syndromes, but in 60% of patients it is X-linked (and thus more common in males). The autosomal recessive form results from deficiency of adenosine deaminase (ADA), an enzyme in purine metabolism.

B. **Acquired immunodeficiency syndrome (AIDS)** is a multisystemic disease caused by human immunodeficiency virus (HIV).

1. **Transmission.** HIV is transmitted via semen and vaginal secretions, blood, and breast milk. Modes of transmission include unprotected sex (genitogenital or anogenital), contaminated needles, and contaminated blood products.

2. Pathogenesis. HIV infects CD4$^+$ cells and macrophages. The CD4$^+$ cells are killed, whereas the macrophages serve as a reservoir for the virus. Lymphopenia resulting from HIV-mediated killing of CD4$^+$ cells lowers the body's resistance to infections.

3. Clinical presentation
  a. The **acute phase (phase I)** occurs 2–4 weeks after infection and presents with symptoms similar to those of any other acute viral syndrome (e.g., fever, fatigue, sore throat, lymphadenopathy).
  b. The **latent phase (phase II)** is of variable duration. During this phase, patients are asymptomatic.
  c. The **late phase (phase III)** is characterized by a decrease in the CD4$^+$ cell count and persistent lymphadenopathy.
  d. The **final crisis (phase IV)** is marked by a general decline in the patient's well-being, the appearance of tumors (e.g., **Kaposi sarcoma, lymphoma, invasive carcinoma** of the cervix or skin), or the development of recurrent infections. Certain infections are considered typical features of AIDS, including:
    (1) Pneumonia caused by *Pneumocystis carinii*, cytomegalovirus (CMV), or herpes simplex virus (HSV)
    (2) Central nervous system (CNS) infections caused by *Toxoplasma gondii* and *Cryptococcus neoformans*
    (3) Gastrointestinal infections caused by *Mycobacterium avium-intracellulare* (MAI), *Candida albicans*, CMV, or *Cryptosporidium* species
    (4) Disseminated infections caused by CMV, HSV, varicella zoster virus, and fungi (e.g., coccidioidomycosis)

V. IMMUNOLOGIC COMPLICATIONS OF ORGAN TRANSPLANTATION.
Transplanted organs usually elicit T-cell and B-cell reactions, targeting primarily the major histocompatibility antigen (MHA) on the surface of graft cells.

A. Transplant rejection

  1. Hyperacute rejection occurs within minutes or hours and results from the attachment of preexisting antibodies to the endothelial cells of the graft, leading to endotheliosis and thrombosis of major vessels.

  2. Acute rejection occurs days, months, or years after transplantation and is mediated either by antibodies or lymphocytes. The humoral (antibody) response is usually characterized by obliterative vasculitis.

  3. Chronic rejection usually occurs after several bouts of acute rejection, from which it differs only in the degree of vascular obliteration.

B. Graft-versus-host disease (GVHD) typically occurs following **bone marrow transplants.** T lymphocytes transplanted with other hematopoietic cells attack the host cells or secrete cytokines that adversely affect the transplant recipient.

  1. Dermatologic manifestations include desquamative dermatitis in the acute phase and sclerosis in the late phase.

  2. Hepatic findings. Bile duct destruction leads to cholestatic jaundice.

  3. Gastrointestinal findings. Epithelial cell necrosis results in malabsorption and bloody diarrhea.

  4. Hematologic findings. Bone marrow involvement leads to suppression of normal hematopoiesis.

4

Neoplasia

I. INTRODUCTION

A. Definition. Neoplasia is the uncontrolled proliferation of cells. Neoplastic masses may be benign (i.e., likely to remain localized) or malignant (i.e., likely to be invasive and metastatic).

> **Although neoplasms are commonly referred to as "tumors," not all tumors are neoplasms! For example, hamartomas are tumor-like masses composed of cells normally found in that particular organ but abnormally arranged.**

B. Histologic/histogenetic classification of neoplasia. Pathologists classify neoplastic masses according to their microscopic features and presumed histogenesis.

1. Mesenchymal (connective tissue) origin
   a. **Benign mesenchymal tumors** are designated by adding the suffix **"-oma"** to the name of the cell that comprises the tumor.

> **Not all tumors ending in "-oma" are benign! Important examples of malignant tumors ending in "-oma" include lymphoma, glioma, melanoma, and seminoma.**

   b. **Malignant mesenchymal tumors** are called **sarcomas** (Table 4-1).

2. Epithelial origin
   a. **Benign epithelial tumors** are called **adenomas, polyps,** or **papillomas.**
   b. **Malignant epithelial tumors** are called **carcinomas** (Table 4-2).

> **Carcinomas form nests of epithelial cells that are separate from the nonneoplastic stroma. This is in contrast to the cells of sarcomas, which are intermixed with the mesenchymal (connective tissue) stroma.**

3. Germ cell origin. **Teratomas** are derived from one or more of the three embryonic germ cell layers:

Table 4-1
Tumors of Mesenchymal Origin

Cell Type	Benign Tumor	Malignant Tumor
Fibroblast	Fibroma	Fibrosarcoma
Fat cell	Lipoma	Liposarcoma
Smooth muscle cell	Leiomyoma	Leiomyosarcoma
Striated muscle cell	Rhabdomyoma	Rhabdomyosarcoma
Bone cell	Osteoma	Osteosarcoma
Endothelial cell	Hemangioma	Angiosarcoma

Table 4-2
Tumors of Epithelial Origin

Type of Epithelium	Benign Tumor	Malignant Tumor
Glandular or ductal cells	Adenoma ("polyp" on mucosal surfaces)	Adenocarcinoma
Transitional cell	Transitional cell papilloma	Transitional cell carcinoma
Squamous cell	Seborrheic keratosis	Squamous cell carcinoma
Organ- or tissue-specific cells	Hepatocellular adenoma, renal cell adenoma	Hepatocellular carcinoma, renal cell carcinoma

    a. Ectoderm gives rise to **skin** and **nervous tissue.**
    b. Mesoderm gives rise to **muscle** and **bone.**
    c. Endoderm gives rise to **intestinal** and **bronchial tissue.**

4. **Specialized tissue or cell origin.** Tumors of specialized tissues or cells are **named according to the type of cell they originated from.** For example, in the brain, one finds gliomas, meningiomas, neurocytomas, and neuroblastomas. In the testis, one finds seminomas (which originate from germ cells), Sertoli cell adenomas, and Leydig cell adenomas.

5. **Uncertain origin.** Tumors of uncertain origin that cannot be classified precisely often have **eponymous names** (e.g., Ewing sarcoma, Hodgkin disease).

II. BIOLOGY OF CANCER.
Malignant neoplastic cells differ from normal cells in many aspects:

    A. **Growth *in vivo*.** In contrast with normal cells, tumor cells:

        1. Invade the basement membranes of tissues, through the action of lytic enzymes

        2. Detach from neighboring cells (i.e., they lack surface adhesion molecules, such as cadherin)

        3. Have the ability to metastasize (i.e., spread via the blood, lymphatic system, or seeding of body cavities)

        4. Exhibit clonal expansion (i.e., the cells originating from a single tumor cell overgrow all others)

        5. Are able to induce angiogenesis

B. **Growth** *in vitro.* In contrast with normal cells, tumor cells:

1. Lack contact inhibition (i.e., they show no growth restriction *in vitro*)

2. Exhibit anchorage-independent growth in soft agar

3. Exhibit growth factor-independent growth (autocrine stimulation)

C. **Dedifferentiation (anaplasia).** In contrast with normal cells, tumor cells exhibit:

1. A loss of specialized functions

2. Simplified cytoplasmic architecture

3. Fetal features and antigens [e.g., α-fetoprotein (AFP) in liver cancer, carcinoembryonic antigen (CEA) in colon cancer]

The degree of dedifferentiation is used for histologic grading of tumors; the extent of spread of the tumor is used for clinical staging.

D. **Pleomorphism.** Tumor cells have:

1. Nuclei of varying size and shape

2. Hyperchromatic nuclei

3. Mitotic abnormalities

4. Chromosomal abnormalities, both structural (e.g., the Philadelphia chromosome in chronic myelogenous leukemia) and numerical (e.g., aneuploidy)

III. CAUSES OF CANCER. The causes of most human cancers are not known, although epidemiologic, genetic, clinical, and laboratory studies have identified many potential causes of cancer.

A. **Chemical carcinogens** are summarized in Table 4-3.

Table 4-3
Chemical Carcinogens

Carcinogen	Associated Cancer
Polycyclic hydrocarbons	Carcinoma of the lung, mouth, esophagus, pancreas, urinary bladder, and cervix
Industrial chemicals	
Aniline dyes	Transitional carcinoma of the bladder
Benzene	Leukemia
Nitrosamines	Esophageal and gastric cancers
Benzanthracene	Skin cancer
Heavy metals and inorganic chemicals	
Arsenic	Skin cancer
Asbestos	Mesotheliomas, lung cancer
Uranium	Lung cancer
Nickel, chromium, cadmium	Lung cancer
Drugs	
Diethylstilbestrol (DES)	Vaginal clear cell carcinoma
Alkylating agents	Leukemia, lymphoma
Cyclophosphamide	Urinary bladder cancer
Natural plant products	
Aflatoxin B	Hepatic cancer
Betel nut	Mouth cancer

B. Physical carcinogens include **ultraviolet light** (e.g., sunshine) and **radiation** (e.g., x-rays, atomic bomb explosions, nuclear power plant accidents).

C. Viral carcinogens are summarized in Table 4-4.

D. Oncogenes are cancer-producing genes derived from normal components of the human genome (i.e., proto-oncogenes). Proto-oncogenes become oncogenes through:

1. Mutation (e.g., the *ras* oncogene, implicated in many cancers)

2. Translocation (e.g., the *abl* oncogene, implicated in leukemia, and the *myc* oncogene, implicated in Burkitt's lymphoma)

3. Amplification (e.g., the N-*myc* oncogene, implicated in neuroblastoma)

4. Overexpression (e.g., the *erb*-b2 oncogene, implicated in breast cancer)

E. Inactivation of tumor suppressor genes. Tumor suppressor genes are genes that prevent cancer formation. Loss or inactivation of these genes leads to neoplastic proliferation of cells. Examples of tumor suppression genes are given in Table 4-5.

F. Defective DNA repair and chromosomal instability syndromes. An increased incidence of lung cancer has been noted in patients with certain autosomal recessive disorders characterized by increased fragility of DNA strands, chromosomes, or both, especially following exposure to ultraviolet rays or x-rays. Other hereditary disorders characterized by defective DNA repair or chromosomal instability include:

1. Xeroderma pigmentosum, which is associated with skin tumors

Table 4-4
Viral Carcinogens

Carcinogen	Associated Cancer
Human T-cell lymphotropic virus-1 (HTLV-1)	Adult T-cell lymphoma and leukemia
Human papilloma virus (HPV)	Squamous cell carcinoma of the cervix, vulva, vagina, anus, and larynx
Herpesvirus-8	Kaposi sarcoma
Epstein-Barr virus (EBV)	Burkitt lymphoma, nasopharyngeal carcinoma
Hepatitis B virus (HBV), hepatitis C virus (HCV)	Hepatocellular carcinoma

Table 4-5
Tumor Suppressor Genes

Gene	Associated Cancer
RB	Retinoblastoma, osteosarcoma
TP53	Gastrointestinal, lung, and CNS tumors
APC	Adenomatous polyposis coli
WT1	Wilms tumor
NF1, NF2	Neurofibromatosis types 1 and 2, respectively
BRCA1, BRCA2	Breast cancer

CNS = central nervous system.

2. Ataxia-teleangiectasia, which is associated with an increased incidence of lymphoma, leukemia, and breast carcinoma

3. Fanconi syndrome, which is associated with an increased incidence of lymphoma and leukemia

4. Bloom syndrome, which is associated with a high incidence of lymphoma and leukemia

IV. EPIDEMIOLOGY OF CANCER. The main epidemiologic parameters used in the study of cancer are sex, age, race, ethnicity, geography, and environmental conditions.

A. Sex

1. Female predominance is seen in **carcinoma of the breast** and **thyroid cancer.**

2. Male predominance is seen in **esophageal cancer** and **pancreatic cancer.**

B. Age. The incidence of most tumors increases with age. Important exceptions include:

1. Retinoblastoma and **Wilms tumor** (peak incidence during childhood)

2. Testicular germ cell tumors (peak incidence between the ages of 25 and 45 years)

3. Hodgkin disease (peak incidence between the ages of 20 and 25 years, and then again at the age of 60 years)

C. Race, ethnicity, and geography

1. Breast cancer. The incidence is lower in Japanese women, as compared with American women.

2. Gastric cancer. The incidence is higher in Japan and Iceland, as compared with the United States.

3. Hepatic cancer. The incidence is higher in sub-Saharan African countries, as compared with the United States.

4. Prostate cancer. In the United States, black men are more likely than white men to develop prostate cancer.

5. Skin cancer is more common in patients with fair skin, light hair, and blue or green eyes.

D. Environmental conditions. Occupation or workplace can predispose the patient to certain cancers. For example:

1. Bladder cancer is seen more often in patients who work in industries involving the manufacture or use of aniline dyes, textiles, or rubber.

2. Mesothelioma is seen more often in patients whose work exposed them to asbestos (e.g., pipefitters, ship builders).

V. EFFECTS OF CANCER

A. Local effects include compression and destruction of normal tissue, obstruction (e.g., of the intestine, bronchi, or bile ducts), erosion of blood vessels, and bone fractures.

B. Cachexia. Weight loss and weakness in patients with cancer has many causes:

1. Anorexia

2. Difficulty on swallowing

3. Malabsorption

4. "Parasitic" usage of nutrients by the tumor

5. Cytokine effects

6. Chemotherapy

C. Paraneoplastic syndromes are symptom complexes seen in patients with cancer that are not caused directly by the mass or its metastases. These symptom complexes are caused by hormones, polypeptides, and immune factors, and have many manifestations. Examples include:

1. Endocrinologic and metabolic disorders (e.g., hypercalcemia, Cushing syndrome, hypoglycemia)

2. Hematologic and vascular disorders (e.g., erythrocytosis, Trousseau syndrome)

3. Neuromuscular disorders (e.g., dermatomyositis, Lambert-Eaton syndrome)

4. Dermatologic disorders (e.g., acanthosis nigricans) *symmetric mm. wkness ↑↑ enzyme levels + skin rash*

5. Renal disorders (e.g., nephrotic syndrome)

VI. DIAGNOSIS OF CANCER

A. Clinical diagnosis encompasses the **history** and **physical examination, radiographic studies,** and **laboratory studies.** Tumor markers are summarized in Table 4-6.

B. Cytology. Cell samples are obtained for analysis via aspiration through a thin needle or via exfoliation (e.g., as in a Pap smear).

C. Biopsy. Tissue samples may be obtained for analysis via a needle or by surgical excision.

1. Standard histologic slides are stained with hematoxylin (stains the nuclei blue) and eosin (stains the cytoplasm red).

2. Immunohistochemistry entails the use of specific antibodies to detect tumor markers.

3. Molecular diagnosis. Techniques include the Southern blot test (to evaluate DNA), the Northern blot test (to evaluate RNA), and the polymerase chain reaction (PCR) test.

4. Flow cytometry is used to analyze and prove the clonality of lymphomas and leukemias.

Table 4-6
Tumor Markers

Marker	Associated Cancer
Hormones	
Human chorionic gonadotropin (hCG)	Choriocarcinoma, teratocarcinoma
Adrenocorticotropic hormone (ACTH)	Small cell carcinoma of the lung
Parathyroid-like polypeptide	Squamous cell carcinoma of the bronchi
Calcitonin	Medullary carcinoma of the thyroid
Oncofetal proteins	
Carcinoembryonic antigen (CEA)	Colon cancer
α-Fetoprotein (AFP)	Hepatocellular carcinoma
Normal proteins	
Monoclonal gammaglobulin	Multiple myeloma
Prostate-specific antigen (PSA)	Prostate carcinoma

5

Developmental and Genetic Diseases

I. DEVELOPMENTAL ANOMALIES

A. Types of developmental anomalies

1. **Agenesis** is failure of an organ to develop (e.g., renal agenesis in Potter syndrome).

2. **Atresia** is obliteration of an organ's lumen (e.g., esophageal atresia).

3. **Hypoplasia** is a smaller-than-normal organ (e.g., microcephaly).

4. **Ectopia** is an abnormally located organ (e.g., cryptorchid testis).

5. **Syndactyly** is fusion of the digits.

B. **Causes of developmental anomalies.** In most cases, the cause of the developmental defect cannot be determined. Proven **teratogens** are given in Table 5-1.

II. CHROMOSOMAL DISORDERS

A. The **normal karyotype** is 46,XX or 46,XY. Each cell has 44 autosomes and 2 sex chromosomes (i.e., XX or XY).

1. The normal karyotype is **euploid** (i.e., it has a full complement of chromosomes).

2. The normal karyotype is **diploid** (i.e., it consists of two complete haploid sets, each containing 23 chromosomes).

Table 5-1
Common Developmental Defects

Cause	Associated Defects
Alcohol	Growth and mental retardation, abnormal facies, various other abnormalities (fetal alcohol syndrome)
Thalidomide	Phocomelia (i.e., foreshortening of the limbs)
DES	Vaginal adenosis
TORCH infection	Brain lesions (e.g., microcephaly, calcifications), cataracts, heart defects (e.g., PDA, septal defects), purpura, liver disease
Treponema pallidum infection (congenital syphilis)	Bone abnormalities (saber shins), malformed teeth, blindness, deafness

DES = diethylstilbestrol; PDA = patent ductus arteriosus.

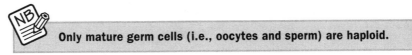

Only mature germ cells (i.e., oocytes and sperm) are haploid.

B. **Karyotype abnormalities** may be **numerical** or **structural.**

1. **Numerical abnormalities**
   a. **Aneuploidy** is an abnormal number of chromosomes that is not a multiple of the normal haploid number. **Monosomy** (one copy of a chromosome) and **trisomy** (three copies of a chromosome) usually result from **nondisjunction** during meiosis (Figure 5–1). Some of the better-known disorders caused by aneuploid errors in the chromosome complement are summarized in Table 5-2.
   b. **Polyploidy** is an abnormal number of chromosomes resulting from the presence of more than two complete haploid sets (e.g., $3 \times 23 = 69$, $4 \times 23 = 92$).

2. **Structural abnormalities**
   a. **Deletion** refers to the loss of a portion of a chromosome. **Cri du chat syndrome** is an example of a disorder caused by deletion.
   b. **Translocation** occurs when a segment of one chromosome is transferred to a nonhomologous chromosome following breakage of both.

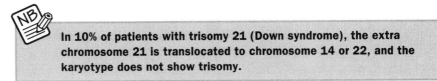

In 10% of patients with trisomy 21 (Down syndrome), the extra chromosome 21 is translocated to chromosome 14 or 22, and the karyotype does not show trisomy.

   c. **Isochromosome.** An isochromosome is an abnormal chromosome with a median centromere and two pairs of identical arms, as opposed to one pair of long arms and one pair of short arms.

III. GENETIC DISORDERS. Single gene defects occur at random in germ cells or embryonic cells. Usually they are either minor and clinically unimportant, or lethal. Those that cause disease may be transmitted to the next generation as hereditary (familial) disorders.

A. **Causes of gene defects.** The cause of most single gene defects is not known, and only a minority of genetic defects can be traced to the effects of viruses, chemicals, or radiation.

B. **Mechanisms of gene defects**

1. **Point mutation.** A single nucleotide is substituted for another one in the coding sequence (e.g., glutamic acid is substituted for valine at locus 6 of the β chains of hemoglobin A in sickle cell anemia). Point mutations can occur in the intron, promoter, or enhancer sequences.

2. **Frameshift mutation.** The deletion or insertion of nucleotides into the coding sequence causes a shift in gene transcription and translation.

C. Methods of inheritance of gene defects

1. **Mendelian inheritance**
   a. **Autosomal dominant**
      (1) **Features of autosomal dominant inheritance**
         (a) Because the gene is located on an autosome, males and females are affected equally.
         (b) The trait is expressed in heterozygotes (Aa) and is therefore found in every generation, including the parents, unless the trait is a new mutation. Fifty percent of the offspring are affected.

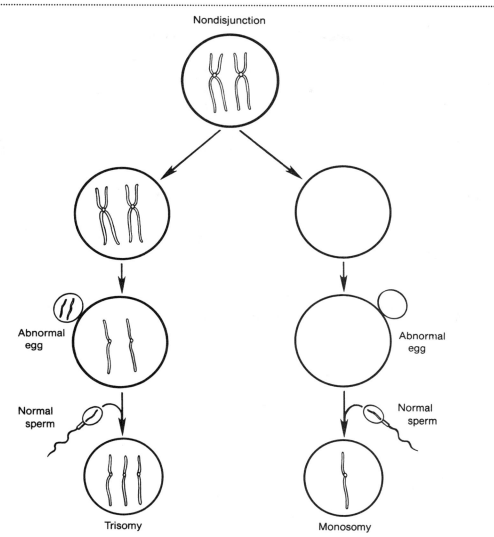

Figure 5-1.   Nondisjunction during meiosis (i.e., the process by which germ cells become haploid), occurring in this case in the oocyte. The unequal distribution of the chromosomes can result in either trisomic (*left*) or monosomic (*right*) zygotes after fertilization by a normal haploid gamete, in this case, the sperm cell. (Reprinted with permission from Johnson KE: *NMS Human Developmental Anatomy*. Baltimore, Williams & Wilkins, 1988, p 27.)

        (c) Children who inherit the gene may not exhibit the trait if the gene has low penetrance or variable expressivity.

    (2) **Autosomal dominant disorders** usually involve genes that code for structural proteins, receptors, or transport proteins.

        (a) Symptoms of most autosomal dominant diseases appear with some latency, and many of these disorders are diagnosed in adulthood (e.g., the dementia of Huntington disease appears at the age of 30–50 years).

        (b) The most important autosomal dominant disorders are listed in Table 5-3 .

Table 5-2.
Chromosomal Disorders Caused by Aneuploidy

Syndrome	Incidence	Clinical Features
Trisomy 21 (Down syndrome)	1:800	Mental retardation, characteristic facial features (i.e., epicanthic folds, macroglossia, flat occiput), simian crease, cardiac defects, increased risk for leukemia
Trisomy XXY (47,XXY; Klinefelter syndrome)*	1:850	Testicular hypoplasia, eunuchoid body habitus, long extremities, high FSH levels and low testosterone levels, absence of secondary sexual characteristics, irreversible infertility (azoospermia)
Monosomy X (45,X; Turner syndrome)†	1:3000	Streak ovaries, webbed neck, short stature, broad chest, coarctation of the aorta, absence of secondary sexual characteristics, primary amenorrhea and infertility
Trisomy 18 (Edward syndrome)	1:8000	Multiple malformations; most patients die in infancy
Trisomy 13 (Patau syndrome)	1:15,000	Multiple malformations; most patients die in infancy

* These patients may have more than two X chromosomes (e.g., karyotype 48,XXXY).
† Only 50% of these patients lack the entire X chromosome and are 45,X. The others are either mosaics (i.e., their bodies are composed of cells lacking the X chromosome as well as cells that have it) or they have an abnormal second X chromosome (e.g., a ring chromosome, isochromosome, or deletion of a long or short arm of the X chromosome).

Table 5-3
Autosomal Dominant Disorders

Neurologic disorders
  Huntington chorea

Musculoskeletal disorders
  Achondroplasia
  Marfan syndrome
  Myotonic dystrophy
  Osteogenesis imperfecta (certain forms)
  Ehlers-Danlos syndrome

Hematopoietic disorders
  Hereditary spherocytosis
  von Willebrand disease

Urinary disorders
  Adult polycystic kidney disease

Metabolic disorders
  Familial hypercholesterolemia

Tumor syndromes
  Neurofibromatosis
  Familial polyposis coli
  Wilms tumor
  Retinoblastoma
  Li-Fraumeni syndrome (i.e., early breast carcinoma associated with soft tissue sarcomas and other tumors)

  b. Autosomal recessive inheritance
   (1) Features of autosomal recessive inheritance
      (a) Because the gene is located on an autosome, males and females are affected equally.
      (b) The trait is expressed only in homozygotes (aa) who have inherited an abnormal allele from each parent. Parents are asymptomatic heterozygotes (Aa) and each of their offspring has a 25% chance of being homozygous for the recessive allele (aa).
   (2) **Autosomal recessive disorders** usually involve genes that code for enzymes.
      (a) The metabolic error usually becomes evident early in life.
      (b) Autosomal recessive disorders, examples of which are given in (Table 5-4), represent the largest group of genetic disorders.
  c. X-linked (sex-linked) inheritance
   (1) Features of X-linked inheritance
      (a) The gene is located on the X chromosome and is donated by the mother, who is asymptomatic. Only sons develop the trait; daughters inherit the gene in 50% of cases and become asymptomatic carriers.
      (b) All daughters of the affected male are asymptomatic carriers. His sons are neither affected nor carriers.
   (2) **X-linked (sex-linked) disorders.** Only the X-linked recessive disorders are of clinical importance, because X-linked dominant disorders are very rare. The most important X-linked recessive disorders are listed in Table 5-5 .
  d. **Exceptions to the general rules of Mendelian inheritance.** Some genes on autosomes and sex chromosomes are not expressed in conformity with the general rules of Mendelian inheritance.
   (1) **Triple nucleotide repeats.** Certain nucleotide triplets on autosomes or X chromosomes may increase in number, disrupting the normal function of the affected gene. Typically, the amplification becomes more prominent in each subsequent generation, and thus the trait becomes more pronounced.
   (2) **Genomic imprinting.** Usually, it makes no difference whether the allele

Table 5-4.
Autosomal Recessive Disorders

Metabolic diseases
  Cystic fibrosis
  Hemochromatosis
  Lysosomal storage diseases
  Albinism
  Phenylketonuria
  Glycogen storage diseases
  Galactosemia

Hematopoietic diseases
  Sickle cell anemia
  Thalassemia major

Neuromuscular diseases
  Friedreich ataxia
  Muscular dystrophy (some forms)

Endocrine diseases
  Congenital adrenal hyperplasia (21-hydroxylase deficiency)

Table 5-5.
X-linked (Sex-Linked) Recessive Disorders

Duchenne muscular dystrophy

Hemophilia A and B

Fragile X syndrome

Bruton agammaglobulinemia

Wiskott-Aldrich syndrome

Lesch-Nyhan syndrome

Glucose-6-phosphate dehydrogenase (G6PD) deficiency

Hunter syndrome

---

is inherited from the mother or the father. However, the expression of some genes (called "imprinted" genes) depends on their origin (i.e., maternal or paternal). For example, the deletion of genes from the paternally derived chromosome 15 results in Prader-Willi syndrome, whereas deletion of the same genes from maternally derived chromosome 15 results in Angelman (happy puppet) syndrome.

2. **Polygenic inheritance** involves multiple genes.
  a. **Features of polygenic inheritance**
    (1) Inheritance is variable, but the risk is the same for all first-degree relatives (2%–7%)
    (2) Concordance among identical twins is 20%–40%.
  b. **Polygenic disorders.** Many common human traits and diseases are multifactorial and polygenic. Important polygenic disorders include hypertension, diabetes mellitus, psychiatric disorders (e.g., manic depression, schizophrenia), congenital heart diseases, cleft lip and palate, and cerebrospinal dysraphic disorders (e.g., anencephaly, spina bifida).

3. **Mitochondrial inheritance.** Mitochondria contain circular DNA molecules (mitochondrial genes), which account for less than 1% of the genome.
  a. Mitochondrial genes are inherited from the mother and passed to both sons and daughters.
  b. These genes encode for the enzymes involved in oxidative phosphorylation; therefore, mutation of these genes affects organs with high energy requirements (e.g., muscles, eyes, CNS structures). Examples of diseases caused by mutations of mitochondrial genes include:
    (1) **Leber hereditary optic neuropathy**
    (2) **Kearns-Sayre syndrome** (characterized by ophthalmoplegia, myopathy, ataxia, and cardiac conduction abnormalities)
    (3) **Myoclonus epilepsy with ragged red fibers (MERRF) syndrome**

6

Hemodynamic Disorders

I. EDEMA is the accumulation of fluid in interstitial spaces or body cavities. Clinically important forms of edema are listed in Table 6-1.

A. Mechanisms of edema

1. Increased intravascular (hydrostatic) pressure can result from impaired venous return or arteriolar dilatation.

2. Reduced plasma oncotic pressure results from hypoalbuminemia. Causes of hypoalbuminemia include nephrotic syndrome, protein-losing enteropathy, and hepatic cirrhosis (which is associated with decreased protein production).

3. Increased interstitial oncotic pressure is caused by sodium retention. Sodium retention is associated with renal failure and congestive heart failure (CHF). In CHF, renal hypoperfusion stimulates the renin–angiotensin system, leading to sodium and water retention by the kidneys.

4. Increased vascular permeability is seen in inflammation.

5. Lymphatic obstruction can result from neoplasia or chronic inflammation.

B. Forms of edema

1. Transudates are caused by increased hydrostatic pressure or reduced plasma oncotic pressure. The fluid has a low protein content (i.e., the specific gravity is less than 1.020), and contains few cells.

2. Exudates are caused by inflammation. The fluid has a high protein content (i.e., the specific gravity is greater than 1.020), and contains numerous inflammatory cells.

II. HYPEREMIA is an increased amount of blood in part of the body.

A. Active hyperemia is the increased influx of arterial blood to a particular area. Physiologic causes of active hyperemia include flushing as a result of exercise, blushing, and inflammation.

B. Passive hyperemia (congestion) is caused by reduced venous outflow. Stasis of poorly oxygenated blood can lead to parenchymal damage.

1. Chronic passive hyperemia of the **liver** in patients with **right ventricular failure** produces a characteristic **"nutmeg liver" pattern** (i.e., multiple small, red, depressed centrolobular areas surrounded by viable parenchyma, which is tan).

Table 6-1
Clinically Important Forms of Edema

Type	Cause
Anasarca (generalized edema)	Nephrotic syndrome
Peripheral edema (pitting leg edema)	CHF, right ventricular failure
Pulmonary edema	Left ventricular failure
Brain edema	Head trauma
Ascites (accumulation of fluid in the peritoneal cavity)	Cirrhosis
Hydrothorax	CHF, pleuritis
Hydropericardium	Viral pericarditis

CHF = congestive heart failure.

   2. Chronic passive hyperemia of the **lungs** in patients with **left ventricular failure** leads to alveolar fibrosis (**"brown induration of the lungs"**) and intra-alveolar hemorrhages. The extravasated red blood cells (RBCs) undergo hemolysis and are taken up by alveolar macrophages. The hemosiderin-laden macrophages are known as **"heart failure cells."**

III. HEMORRHAGE is the escape of blood from the circulatory system. Hemorrhage may be **internal** (leading to the accumulation of blood in the tissues, body cavities, or lumens of internal organs) or **external.** Common clinical manifestations of internal hemorrhage are summarized in Table 6-2.

   A. Hematomas are localized collections of blood (usually clotted) in tissue.

   B. Hemothorax, hemopericardium, and **hemoperitoneum** are terms used to describe hemorrhage in body cavities (i.e., the thoracic, pericardial, and the peritoneal cavities, respectively).

IV. THROMBOSIS. Thrombogenesis, the process common to both hemostasis (i.e., normal blood clot formation) and thrombosis, depends on endothelial cells, platelets, and plasma coagulation proteins.

   A. Hemostasis is physiologic blood clotting. Injury to the endothelium-lined vessel wall initiates a four-phase process:

   1. Vasoconstriction. Arteriolar smooth muscle cells react to neurogenic stimuli and **endothelin,** a potent vasoconstrictor secreted by endothelial cells.

   2. Hemostatic plug formation (primary hemostasis). Platelets are attracted to the subendothelial extracellular matrix, which was exposed by the injury. The **platelets** adhere to the extracellular matrix (a process mediated by **von Willebrand factor**), change shape, and release secretory granules (e.g., **thromboxane A_2**). These secretory granules recruit more platelets (a process called **aggregation**).

   3. Fibrin clot formation (secondary hemostasis)
      a. Activation of the coagulation cascade leads to **fibrin deposition.** Eventually, the fibrin polymerizes, forming a **meshwork.**
         (1) The **intrinsic pathway** is activated by **platelet factor 3,** which is expressed on the surface of the platelets.
         (2) The **extrinsic pathway** is activated by **tissue factor,** which is released from the damaged tissue.
      b. The **activation of thrombin** during the coagulation sequence leads to further

Table 6-2.
Common Clinical Manifestations of Internal Hemorrhage

Skin, mucosae, or serosal surfaces
Petechiae (pinpoint-sized lesions)
Ecchymoses (bruises)
Purpura (systemic disease characterized by numerous petechiae and ecchymoses)

Gastrointestinal tract
Hematemesis (blood in the vomitus)
Hematochezia (fresh blood in the stool)
Melena (blackened blood in the stool, caused by exposure of blood to hydrochloric acid in the stomach)

Respiratory tract
Epistaxis (nosebleed)
Hemoptysis (expectoration of blood)

Genitourinary tract
Metrorrhagia (excessive uterine bleeding)
Hematuria (blood in the urine)

aggregation of platelets. Thrombin, which binds to the platelet surface, causes platelet contraction **(viscous metamorphosis),** thereby sealing the clot and making it permanent.

4. **Thrombolysis.** Several mediators limit clot formation and participate in dissolution of the clot.
   a. **Tissue plasminogen activator (t-PA),** released from endothelial cells, generates **plasmin.** Plasmin cleaves fibrin into fibrin split products, causing dissolution of the clot.
   b. **Antithrombin III** inactivates thrombin and several coagulation factors (e.g., factor Xa).
   c. **Proteins S** and **C** work together to inhibit clotting by disabling factors Va and VIIa.

B. **Thrombosis** is the pathologic formation of a **blood clot (thrombus)** within the vascular system.

   1. **Thrombus formation.** Three factors **(Virchow's triad)** predispose to inappropriate thrombus formation.
      a. **Endothelial injury** plays a particularly important role in thrombus formation in the cardiac chambers (e.g., following infarction) and arteries (e.g., atherosclerosis).
      b. **Blood flow disturbances** (i.e., **turbulence** and **stasis**) predispose to thrombosis in dilated veins or arterial aneurysms.
      c. **Hypercoagulability** may be seen in association with certain tumors, following surgery, or in patients with congenital coagulopathies.

> **Remember the five "T" risk factors for thrombosis:**
> **Turbulent blood flow**
> **Trauma**
> **Tumors (especially gastrointestinal and pancreatic carcinomas)**
> **Toxins (e.g., bacterial endotoxins)**
> **Treatment (e.g., surgery, postoperative prolonged bed rest, certain medications)**

2. Fate of the thrombus. If not immediately fatal to the patient, thrombi undergo some combination of the following changes over a period of time:
  a. Lysis (i.e., removal by fibrinolytic activity)
  b. Propagation (i.e., accumulation of additional platelets and fibrin)
  c. Organization and recanalization (i.e., the ingrowth of granulation tissue from the vessel wall and the reestablishment of blood flow through the thrombus)
  d. Embolization (i.e., part or all of the thrombus is dislodged from its original site and carried to a distant site within the vascular system)
  e. Infection (i.e., bacterial seeding)

3. Types of thrombi
  a. Arterial thrombi are usually superimposed on atherosclerotic lesions.
    (1) Infarction (ischemic necrosis) is the result of sudden arterial occlusion.
    (2) Chronic ischemia results from slowly progressive occlusions.
  b. Venous thrombi (red thrombi, stasis thrombi) tend to form in slow-moving blood and therefore contain a high number of enmeshed RBCs, hence the designation "red."
    (1) Venous thrombi are seen most often in the **lower extremities,** leading to **venous congestion.** Clinical manifestations include stasis dermatitis and skin ulcers.
    (2) Occlusive thrombi in the **intestinal veins** cause **hemorrhagic (red) infarction.**
  c. Microvascular thrombi are seen in disseminated intravascular coagulation (DIC), a complication of shock, severe infection, cancer, and many other disorders that are associated with the activation of thrombin.
  d. Mural cardiac thrombi are attached to the walls of the cardiac chambers, and often develop over areas of myocardial infarction.
  e. Valvular cardiac thrombi usually are the result of damage to the valves caused by infective endocarditis, but may be sterile in patients with nonbacterial thrombotic endocarditis.

V. EMBOLISM is the intravascular transfer of a solid, liquid, or gaseous mass from one site to another. Eventually, the mass lodges in a vessel that is too narrow to permit its passage, leading to occlusion.

  A. Thromboemboli are the most common type of emboli.

    1. Venous thromboemboli originate in veins and typically lodge in the **lungs.**

    2. Arterial thromboemboli. Most arterial thromboemboli originate from mural thrombi in the left atrium, left ventricle, or aorta, or from mitral and aortic valve vegetations. These emboli may occlude any artery, leading to infarction. The most common clinically important occlusions include those of the **cerebral, intestinal, and renal arteries,** as well as those of the **arteries that supply the lower extremities.**

    3. Paradoxical emboli originate in the veins but pass into the arterial circulation through an open foramen ovale or another septal defect.

  B. Fat emboli are derived from bone marrow and are most often seen following fracture of the long bones. Pulmonary symptoms, neurologic symptoms, and thrombocytopenia develop 1–3 days after the fracture.

  C. Air emboli. Air bubbles can enter the circulation as a result of thoracic trauma, a surgical procedure, or decompression sickness.

  D. Amniotic fluid emboli. The entry of amniotic fluid into the uterine veins is a rare com-

Table 6-3

Pathologic Findings in Shock

Organ	Pathologic Findings
Liver	Centrilobular congestion and necrosis
Kidneys	Acute tubular necrosis
Intestines	Mucosal petechiae, foci of necrosis
Lungs	Edema, hemorrhage, hyaline membranes
Heart	Subendocardial infarction
Brain	Edema and focal ischemic changes

plication of pregnancy that may result in death (owing to occlusion of the pulmonary vessels) or DIC (as a result of thromboplastin in the amniotic fluid).

E. Particulate emboli. Particulate matter—such as cholesterol crystals (from atheromas), bone marrow (from fractured bones), talc (mixed with illicit drugs), and tumor cells— can act as emboli.

VI. SHOCK results when the blood volume is not sufficient to occupy the vascular space, ultimately leading to hypoperfusion and hypoxia of vital organs and multiple organ failure (Table 6-3) .

A. Types of shock

1. Cardiogenic shock ("pump failure") is caused by heart failure (e.g., as a result of myocardial infarction).

2. Hypovolemic shock is caused by massive fluid loss (e.g., as a result of trauma, hemorrhage, or severe burns).

3. Septic (endotoxic) shock is caused by bacterial endotoxins, which induce the release of cytokines. The cytokines, in turn, cause dilatation and increased permeability of the microvasculature (leading to peripheral pooling of blood) and activate the coagulation cascade, leading to DIC.

B. Clinical stages of shock

1. Early, reversible shock. Patients exhibit tachypnea and tachycardia, but their blood pressure is normal.

2. Progressive shock. Patients are in cardiopulmonary distress. Their renal output is decreased and they are hypotensive. Acidosis is noted.

3. Irreversible shock is signaled by multiple organ failure.

7

Pathology of the Cardiovascular System

I. HYPERTENSION is consistent elevation of the systolic or diastolic blood pressure; the generally accepted threshold is any pressure greater than 140/90 mm Hg. Hypertension affects more than 50 million people in the United States.

  A. Causes

    1. Primary (essential) hypertension accounts for 90% of cases of hypertension, and the **cause is unknown.**

    2. Secondary hypertension

      a. Renal disease is the most common cause of secondary hypertension. The release of renin stimulates angiotensin and aldosterone secretion and leads to sodium and water retention.

      b. Endocrine disorders. Hypertension is most often related to **adrenal diseases** (e.g., Cushing syndrome, pheochromocytoma) and **hyperthyroidism.**

      c. Central nervous system (CNS) disorders that are associated with an increased intracranial pressure (ICP), such as a brain tumor, can lead to hypertension.

      d. Pregnancy. Hypertension in pregnancy is multifactorial and may be a sign of preeclampsia!

  B. Pathologic findings

    1. Left ventricular hypertrophy is caused by an increased workload.

    2. Arteriolosclerosis, which presents as hyalinization of the arterioles in benign (typical) hypertension and as hyperplastic obliterative arteriolitis in malignant (accelerated) hypertension, leads to tissue ischemia and is most often seen in the kidneys.

    3. Atherosclerosis (see II) is accelerated by hypertension.

    4. Chronic passive congestion of the lungs, liver, and spleen and **pitting edema** of the lower extremities results from heart failure.

II. ATHEROSCLEROSIS is a multifactorial degenerative disease characterized by the formation of **plaques (atheromas)** on the intima of the blood vessels. Atherosclerosis can cause many clinical syndromes, including **ischemic heart disease, cerebrovascular disease** (e.g., stroke, multi-infarct dementia), **aortic aneurysms, peripheral vascular disease,** and **nephroangiosclerosis** (characterized by hypertension and progressive loss of kidney function).

  A. Risk factors

1. Age greater than 45 years in men, or 55 years in women

2. Male gender

3. **Family history of atherosclerosis** (may be linked to diseases such as familial hypercholesterolemia)

4. **Lipid-rich diet**

5. Hypertension

6. Diabetes

7. Cigarette smoking

B. Pathologic findings

1. **Subendothelial fatty streaks** and **intimal fibrosis** are early lesions.

2. **Atheromas,** plaques consisting of cholesterol-rich debris encased by a fibrous cap, are the **defining lesion** of atherosclerosis. Over time, atheromas undergo changes resulting in **complicated plaques:**

    a. **Occlusive atheroma.** The lesion occludes most of the artery's lumen, leading to tissue ischemia. For example, when the coronary arteries are affected, angina or congestive heart failure (CHF) is the clinical result.

    b. **Ruptured atheroma.** Fissures of the fibrous cap and defects of the endothelial lining cause **thrombosis** or **embolization.**

The formation of an occlusive thrombus over a ruptured atheroma is the most common cause of myocardial infarction. Removal of the thrombus by coronary angioplasty or the administration of tissue plasminogen activator (t-PA) may save the patient's life!

    c. **Weakening of the tunica media** as a result of the atheroma can lead to aneurysm. The abdominal aorta is most often affected.

III. ISCHEMIC HEART DISEASE. Atherosclerosis of the coronary arteries leads to three main clinical syndromes: angina pectoris, myocardial infarction, and CHF.

A. **Angina pectoris** is precordial pain of sudden onset related to hypoperfusion of the myocardium. Most patients with angina pectoris have atherosclerotic narrowing of the coronary arteries.

1. **Types of angina pectoris**

    a. **Prinzmetal (variant) angina** is caused by coronary artery spasm; attacks occur during rest.

    b. **Stable angina** (the most common form of angina pectoris) is related to coronary artery narrowing, which impedes blood flow to the myocardium. Precipitants include excessive or strenuous activity.

    c. **Unstable (crescendo) angina** is caused by platelet thrombi, which lead to the formation of fibrin thrombi and worsening coronary artery stenosis. Unstable angina usually begins as stable angina, but the attacks occur more often and last longer; infarction is usually imminent.

Aspirin inhibits the formation of platelet thrombi and may prevent ischemic heart disease!

2. Pathologic findings

    a. In Prinzmetal angina and stable angina, the myocardium shows no pathologic changes.

    b. In unstable angina, fibrosis replaces dead myocytes.

B. Myocardial infarction is ischemic necrosis of the myocardium.

    1. Types of myocardial infarction. Myocardial infarcts may be either **transmural** or **subendocardial** (Figure 7-1).

    2. Pathologic findings. Necrosis evokes a polymorphonuclear neutrophil (PMN) response 1–3 days after infarction. Macrophages replace the PMNs after 3–7 days. Granulation tissue forms 2–3 weeks after infarction and is eventually replaced by fibrous scar tissue (4–6 weeks after infarction).

        a. Microscopic signs. Dead cells become evident 20–24 hours after the infarction.

        b. Macroscopic changes include **pallor,** followed by **yellowing** (as a result of pus from the PMN response), a **red ring around the periphery** of the necrotic tis-

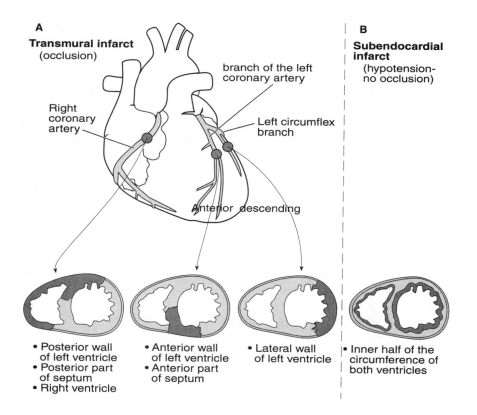

A
Transmural infarct
(occlusion)

branch of the left coronary artery

Right coronary artery

Left circumflex branch

Anterior descending

B
Subendocardial infarct
  (hypotension-
   no occlusion)

• Posterior wall of left ventricle
• Posterior part of septum
• Right ventricle

• Anterior wall of left ventricle
• Anterior part of septum

• Lateral wall of left ventricle

• Inner half of the circumference of both ventricles

Figure 7-1. Types of myocardial infarcts. (A) Transmural infarcts, the most common type, are caused by thrombotic occlusion of a coronary artery. Infarction is localized to the anatomic area supplied by the affected artery. The anterior descending branch of the left coronary artery is affected in 50% of cases. (B) Subendocardial infarcts are circumferential necrosis of the subendocardial myocardium as a result of hypotension (e.g., shock).

sue (as a result of a subsequent attempt at reperfusion), **mottling** (the appearance of the granulation tissue), and **white scarring.**

3. **Clinical diagnosis.** Initially, patients may experience pain and arrhythmias (90% of patients), pulmonary edema owing to heart failure (90% of patients), cardiogenic shock (20%–60% of patients), or sudden death (20% of patients).

   a. **Laboratory findings.** Enzymes, such as creatine kinase (CK), and proteins, such as troponin I, are released from the dying myocytes and can be detected in the patient's blood.

   b. **Electrocardiographic findings** depend on the type of infarct but usually can be detected 6–8 hours after the infarction.

      (1) **Transmural infarcts** show **Q wave changes.**

      (2) **Subendocardial infarcts** do not show Q wave changes.

4. **Complications of myocardial infarction**

   a. **Hemopericardium.** Rupture of the free ventricular wall can lead to hemopericardium. This complication is seen most often during the first week.

   b. **Arterial emboli** may arise from mural thrombi.

   c. **Pericarditis** is seen only in association with transmural myocardial infarction.

   d. **Ventricular aneurysm** is a late complication that usually develops at the site of a large post-infarction scar. The scar tissue does not contract and tends to bulge during systole. A mural thrombus is often present at the site.

   e. **Dressler syndrome (post-myocardial infarction syndrome),** a late complication, is characterized by an autoimmune pericarditis.

IV. INFLAMMATORY HEART DISEASE. Inflammation of the heart may be caused by immune mechanisms or infections. Inflammation may present as **endocarditis, myocarditis,** or **pericarditis,** or it may involve the entire heart **(pancarditis).**

A. **Rheumatic carditis (rheumatic fever)** is an immune-mediated disease that occurs in response to streptococcal antigens, usually following a bout of "strep throat."

   1. **Pathologic findings**

      a. **Verrucous endocarditis** (i.e., wart-like lesions on the valve leaflets) is seen on the mitral and aortic valves. These lesions are sterile.

      b. **Aschoff bodies,** most often found in the myocardium, consist of an area of fibrinoid necrosis surrounded by macrophages.

      c. **Pericarditis.** A sterile fibrinous pericarditis with a "bread and butter" appearance may be seen.

   2. **Clinical diagnosis** is based on the Jones criteria (Table 7-1). The diagnosis is made by documenting an increased anti-streptolysin O (ASO) titer in the presence of either two major criteria or one major and two minor criteria.

   3. **Complications of rheumatic carditis**

      a. **Infectious endocarditis.** The verrucae become infected with bacteria, most often *Streptococcus* species.

      b. **Embolization.** Fibrin verrucae detach and embolize to the brain and other organs.

      c. **Valvular stenosis.** Narrowing results from fibrosis and calcification of the damaged valve. Valvular stenosis is most often seen in the mitral and aortic valves.

      d. **Valvular insufficiency.** Fibrosis and calcification prevent the valve from closing, leading to the regurgitation of blood.

         (1) **Mitral insufficiency** leads to the backflow of blood from the left ventricle into the left atrium during systole.

Table 7-1
Jones Criteria

Major Criteria	Minor Criteria
Polyarthritis	Fever
Carditis	Elevated erythrocyte sedimentation rate (ESR)
Chorea	Leukocytosis
Erythema induratum (subcutaneous nodules)	Prolonged PR interval on EKG
Erythema marginatum	History of rheumatic fever or rheumatic heart disease

EKG = electrocardiogram.

(2) **Aortic insufficiency** leads to the backflow of blood from the aorta to the left ventricle during diastole.

e. **Constrictive pericarditis.** Resolution of the pericarditis causes obliteration of the pericardial sac.

B. **Infective endocarditis** is usually caused by bacteria, but may be caused by fungi in immunosuppressed patients. *Streptococcus* and *Staphylococcus* species account for more than 80% of cases of infective endocarditis.

 Viruses do not cause endocarditis!

1. Predisposing factors
   a. Rheumatic endocarditis
   b. Congenital defects [e.g., bicuspid aortic valve, ventricular septal defect (VSD)]
   c. Therapeutic interventions (e.g., prosthetic valves, indwelling catheters)
   d. Sepsis

2. Pathologic findings
   a. **Valvular endocarditis.** Small excrescences, usually on the mitral and aortic valves, develop into large, friable lesions that may obstruct the valve orifice.
   b. **Mural endocarditis.** Excrescences are typically found on congenital defects (e.g., VSD) or on thrombi overlying an infarct.

3. Complications of infective endocarditis
   a. **Valve destruction.** Bacteria invade the valves, leading to ulceration, rupture, or perforation of the valve.
   b. **Septic emboli.** Thromboemboli carrying bacteria cause infarcts, which become infected and transform into abscesses.
   c. **Immune complex formation and deposition (type III hypersensitivity reactions)** primarily affects the kidneys (glomerulonephritis).
   d. **Persistent sepsis.** The vegetations are a constant source of bacteria, which can be recovered on blood culture.

C. **Myocarditis** is inflammation of the myocardium.

1. **Causes.** Myocarditis may be infectious in origin, immune mediated, or idiopathic.
   a. Most often, the cause is not identified.

    b. Most infections are viral (e.g., coxsackievirus), but in South America, Chagas disease (caused by the protozoon *Trypanosoma cruzi*) is the predominant cause of myocarditis.

  2. **Pathologic findings.** The myocardium is infiltrated with lymphocytes and plasma cells, which are replaced by fibrosis in chronic disease.

  3. **Clinical diagnosis.** Myocarditis should be suspected when heart failure occurs suddenly and without preexisting atherosclerosis.

D. **Pericarditis** is inflammation of the two layers of the pericardial sac (i.e., the epicardium and the pericardium).

  1. **Types of pericarditis.** There are many types of pericarditis, including:
    a. **Infectious pericarditis,** most often caused by viruses or bacteria
    b. **Immune-mediated pericarditis,** such as that seen in rheumatic carditis
    c. **Postinfarction pericarditis,** which results from the inflammatory response to necrosis involving the epicardium in a transmural infarct
    d. **Uremic pericarditis,** a complication of end-stage renal disease (uremia) that may be caused by chemical irritation of the pericardium
    e. **Postsurgical pericarditis** (any heart surgery requires opening of the pericardial sac!)
    f. **Neoplastic pericarditis** (although metastases to the heart are rare, when they occur, they most often involve the epicardium)

  2. **Pathologic findings**
    a. **Serous pericarditis,** the most common form of pericarditis, typically presents as hydropericardium.
    b. **Serofibrinous pericarditis** presents with a fibrin-rich pericardial exudate ("bread and butter" pericarditis).
    c. **Suppurative pericarditis** presents with a purulent exudate.
    d. **Fibrosing pericarditis,** a late complication of other forms of pericarditis, causes cardiac constriction.

  3. **Clinical diagnosis.** Clinically, pericarditis is recognized by a **pericardial friction rub.** Symptoms result from the external compression of the heart.

V. **CARDIOMYOPATHY** is a term used to describe primary noninflammatory disease of the myocardium. The only therapy for cardiomyopathy is cardiac transplantation. Three major clinicopathologic forms are recognized (Figure 7-2).

A. **Dilated cardiomyopathy.** Progressive hypertrophy and dilatation of all four chambers leads to **systolic failure** (i.e., the heart cannot contract). The cause is usually unknown, but viral myocarditis, drugs (e.g., doxorubicin), alcohol, and hemochromatosis may be implicated in some cases.

B. **Hypertrophic cardiomyopathy.** Hypertrophy of the ventricular myocardium leads to **diastolic failure** (i.e., the ventricles cannot dilate). In many cases, the cause of the disease is a genetic disorder that affects myosin and other proteins involved in the contraction of cardiac myocytes.

> **Hypertrophic cardiomyopathy is a rare disease but it is a common cause of sudden death in athletes.**

C. **Restrictive cardiomyopathy,** the rarest type of cardiomyopathy, is characterized by noncompliance of the ventricles, leading to **diastolic failure.** Restrictive cardiomy-

A. Normal

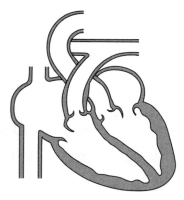

B. Dilated cardiomyopathy

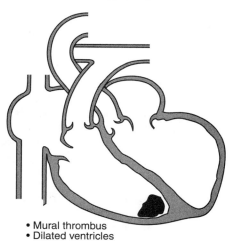

• Mural thrombus
• Dilated ventricles

C. Hypertrophic cardiomyopathy

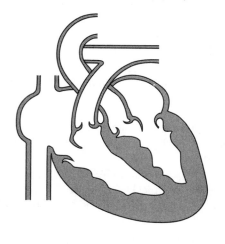

• Asymmetrically thickened septum
• Hypertrophy of the ventricular myocardium

D. Restrictive cardiomyopathy

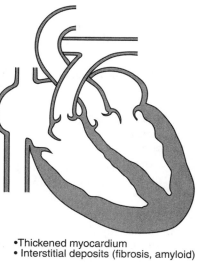

•Thickened myocardium
• Interstitial deposits (fibrosis, amyloid)

Figure 7-2. The three major clinicopathologic forms of cardiomyopathy. (Modified with permission from Damjanov I: *Histopathology A Color Atlas and Textbook*. Baltimore, Williams & Wilkins, 1996, p 108.)

opathy may be caused by fibrosis of the endomyocardium, such as that seen in Löffler endomyocarditis, amyloidosis, and following irradiation.

VI. CONGENITAL HEART DISEASE. The incidence of congenital heart defects is 7 per 1000 live births. The most common congenital heart defects are listed in Table 7-2.

A. Isolated septal defects

    1. Ventricular septal defect (VSD) most often involves the membranous (subvalvular) septum, but may involve the muscular septum as well. Initially, a left-to-right shunt is present, but when the pulmonary pressure increases, the shunt becomes a right-to-left shunt and the patient becomes cyanotic. Blood flow through the shunt produces a holosystolic murmur.

    2. Atrial septal defect (ASD). Three types of ASD are recognized: **ostium secundum ASD** (the most common type), **ostium primum ASD,** and **sinus venosus ASD.** In most patients, ASD is asymptomatic, but the defect may ultimately cause heart failure or serve as a conduit for paradoxical emboli.

B. Stenosis of the great vessels

    1. Aortic or **pulmonary stenosis** causes left or right ventricular hypertrophy, dilatation, and ultimately failure.

    2. Coarctation of the aorta (i.e., narrowing in the region of the aortic arch) is characterized by high pressure in the arteries arising from the aorta proximal to the stenosis (e.g., in the carotid and brachial arteries) and low pressure in the arteries below the stenosis (e.g., the arteries of the lower extremity). Typically, the intercostal arteries act as collateral arteries and supply the thoracic aorta.

C. **Patent ductus arteriosus (PDA).** The ductus arteriosus is a normal fetal vessel that connects the pulmonary artery with the aorta, enabling venous blood to bypass the lungs. Failure of the ductus arteriosus to involute during the first few postnatal days allows backflow of blood from the aorta into the pulmonary artery, producing a "machinery murmur" and causing pulmonary hypertension.

D. **Tetralogy of Fallot** consists of VSD, dextroposition of the aorta, pulmonary stenosis,

Table 7-2
Common Congenital Heart Defects

Defect	Percent Occurrence
Acyanotic defects*	
Ventricular septal defect (VSD)	30
Patent ductus arteriosus (PDA)	10
Pulmonary stenosis	10
Aortic stenosis	10
Coarctation of the aorta	5
Atrial septal defect (ASD)	5
Cyanotic defects	
Tetralogy of Fallot	10
Transposition of the great vessels	5

Modified with permission from Moller JH, Anderson RC: 1,000 consecutive children with a cardiac malformation with 26- to 37-year follow-up. *Am J Cardiol* 70(6):661, 1992.
*Acyanotic defects may progress to cyanotic defects.

and right ventricular hypertrophy (Figure 7-3). Dextroposition of the aorta (i.e., displacement of the aorta to the right) causes the aortic valve to cover the VSD and allows the aorta to receive blood from both the right and left ventricles (i.e., both venous and arterial blood).

1. **Clinical diagnosis.** Entry of venous blood into the aorta results in cyanosis ("blue baby"), easy fatigability early in life, and clubbing of the fingers.

2. **Therapy.** Most patients die during infancy or childhood if the defect is not corrected surgically.

E. Transposition of the great vessels. The aorta originates from the right ventricle and the pulmonary artery originates from the left atrium.

VII. VASCULITIS is a general term for several inflammatory diseases involving blood vessels.

A. Infectious vasculitis

1. **Syphilis.** In tertiary syphilis, inflammation of the vasa vasorum of the aorta (**syphilitic aortitis**) predisposes the patient to aneurysms of the arch of aorta; **meningovascular inflammation** causes tabes dorsalis paralysis and dementia ("general paresis of the insane").

2. **Rickettsial disease** (e.g., Rocky Mountain spotted fever, typhus). The associated vasculitis usually involves the small vessels and is best appreciated on the skin, where it presents as purpura.

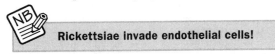
Rickettsiae invade endothelial cells!

3. **Septic emboli.** Bacteria invade the walls of small arteries, leading to mycotic aneurysms or infected infarcts.

B. Autoimmune vasculitis. Several clinicopathologic entities are recognized (Table 7-3).

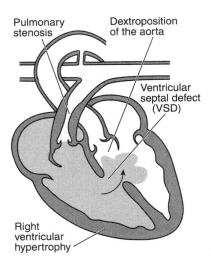

Pulmonary stenosis

Dextroposition of the aorta

Ventricular septal defect (VSD)

Right ventricular hypertrophy

Figure 7-3. Tetralogy of Fallot.

Table 7-3
Types of Autoimmune Vasculitis

Vasculitis	Affected Vessels	Pathologic Findings	Clinical Characteristics
Temporal (giant cell) arteritis	Small arteries, especially the carotids and ocular arteries	Localized granulomatous giant cell reaction	Affects the elderly exclusively; slowly progressive
Polyarteritis nodosa	Small to medium-sized arteries	Type III hypersensitivity reaction with fibrinoid necrosis	Affects adult males most often; may be related to HBV infection
Wegener granulomatosis	Small to medium-sized arteries of the upper respiratory tract, lungs, and kidneys	Necrotizing granulomas of the respiratory tract, necrotizing or granulomatous vasculitis, necrotizing (often crescentic) glomerulonephritis	Average age of onset is 40 years; c-ANCA test positive in 80% of cases
Microscopic polyangiitis (hypersensitivity vasculitis)	Venules, capillaries, and arterioles of the skin, mucous membranes, lungs, heart, gastro-intestinal tract, kidneys, and muscle	Leukocytoclastic destruction of the vessels and focal bleeding; often associated with glomerulonephritis	Presents with nonblanching purpura; often related to drug hypersensitivity; p-ANCA test positive in 80% of cases
Thromboangiitis obliterans (Buerger disease)	Medium-sized vessels of the extremities, especially the radial and tibial arteries	Segmental vasculitis with thrombosis; may spread to adjacent veins and venules	Affects patients who smoke

ANCA = antineutrophil cytoplasm antibody; HBV = hepatitis B virus.

VIII. ANEURYSMS AND VARICES

A. **Aneurysms** are dilatations of the aorta and other arteries that develop where there is significant weakening of the vessel wall.

   1. **Atherosclerotic aneurysms** most often affect the abdominal aorta.

   2. **Syphilitic aneurysms** most often occur in the aortic arch.

   3. **Congenital aneurysms** include **berry aneurysms** (i.e., saccular dilatations of the cerebral artery, usually in the circle of Willis).

   4. **Aortic dissection** (formerly called **dissecting aneurysm**) is dissection of blood between the layers of the arterial wall, leading to rupture of the vessel and massive hemorrhage. Predisposing factors include hypertension and atherosclerosis (in elderly patients) and connective tissue disorders that affect the aorta, such as Marfan syndrome (in younger patients).

   5. **Mycotic aneurysms** are caused by the growth of bacteria in the vessel wall.

B. **Varices (varicosities, varicose veins)** are dilatations of the veins. Clinically, the most important types of varices are varicose veins of the lower extremities, hemorrhoids, and esophageal varices.

8

Pathology of the Respiratory System

I. ATELECTASIS is collapse of the alveoli (in adults) or incomplete expansion of the alveoli (in neonates). The result of atelectasis is reduction of the respiratory surface and hypoxia. Four types of atelectasis are recognized (Figure 8-1).

A. Microatelectasis is a generalized inability of the lung to expand owing to the loss of surfactant.

1. In premature newborns, microatelectasis is seen in **neonatal respiratory distress syndrome** (i.e., incomplete expansion of the lungs of premature infants resulting from the inability of immature type II alveolar cells to secrete surfactant). Gas exchange in the alveolar ducts and respiratory bronchioles leads to cell injury and the deposition of a fibrin exudate, which forms **hyaline membranes** in the alveoli, alveolar ducts, and bronchioles.

2. In adults, microatelectasis may be the result of **adult respiratory distress syndrome (ARDS).** ARDS is a clinical term for diffuse alveolar damage leading to respiratory failure that does not respond to oxygen inhalation. ARDS is associated with a mortality rate of approximately 50%.

a. Causes. ARDS results from injury of either the alveolar or the capillary endothelial cells (i.e., the cells that form the alveolar septa). Typical causes of such injuries are:

(1) Shock. Endotoxins or ischemia can injure the endothelial cells, leading to "leaky capillary syndrome" and disseminated intravascular coagulation (DIC).

(2) Inhalation of toxic gases or **extremely hot air,** which can damage the alveolar cells

(3) Illicit drugs (e.g., **heroin**)

(4) Metabolic disorders (e.g., **uremia, acidosis, acute pancreatitis**)

b. Pathologic findings include intraalveolar edema and hemorrhage, hyaline membranes, and focal atelectasis.

B. Compression atelectasis is mechanical collapse of alveoli owing to external pressure. Compression atelectasis may be caused by pleural effusions, pneumothorax, or a tumor in the pleural space.

C. Resorption atelectasis is collapse of the alveoli distal to an obstructed bronchus. Causes of resorption atelectasis include foreign bodies, mucous plugs (such as those seen in patients with asthma or following surgery), and tumors.

D. Contraction atelectasis is a focal loss of alveoli resulting from interstitial fibrosis. The fibrosis prevents complete expansion and increases elastic recoil.

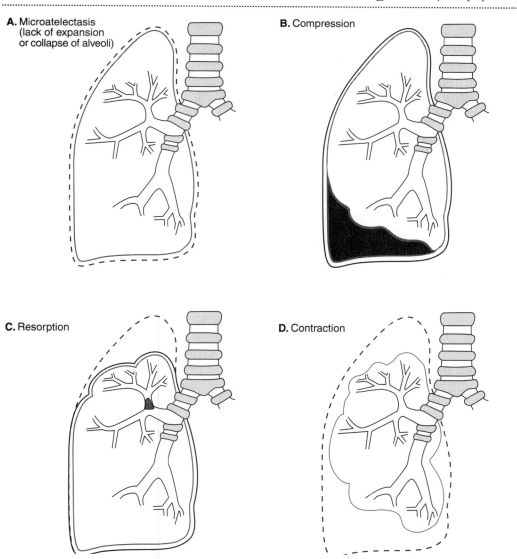

A. Microatelectasis (lack of expansion or collapse of alveoli)

B. Compression

C. Resorption

D. Contraction

Figure 8-1.   Forms of atelectasis. (Redrawn with permission from Kumar V, Cotran RS, Robbins SL: *Basic Pathology*, 6th ed. Philadelphia, WB Saunders, 1997, p 394.)

II. BRONCHIECTASIS is chronic dilatation of the bronchi secondary to obstruction or persistent infection, both of which result in destruction of the smooth muscles and supportive tissues in the wall of the bronchi. Typical causes of bronchiectasis include:

   A. Bronchial obstruction. The bronchi may be obstructed by tumors, foreign bodies, or mucous plugs.

   B. Persistent lung infections. Infections that do not heal or that often recur are found in congenital conditions, such as cystic fibrosis, Kartagener (immotile cilia) syndrome, and immunodeficiency disorders.

III. OBSTRUCTIVE LUNG DISEASES are characterized physiologically by an increased resistance to air flow. The obstruction can occur in the larynx (e.g., acute laryngitis, "croup"), the bronchi (e.g., asthma, chronic bronchitis), the respiratory bronchioles [e.g., bronchiolitis obliterans obstructive pneumonia (BOOP)], or the alveoli (e.g., emphysema).

A. **Asthma,** a chronic inflammatory disease associated with hyperactivity of the bronchi and bronchioles, is characterized by recurrent attacks of bronchospasm and excessive mucus production.

1. Types of asthma
   a. **Atopic asthma** results from an immune response to exogenous allergens. Attacks are mediated initially by IgE, and then by leukotrienes. Children are affected most often.
      (1) The disorder is often familial and associated with atopic dermatitis.
      (2) Usually, atopic asthma resolves spontaneously (i.e., the child "grows out of it"). It rarely causes chronic bronchitis or emphysema.
   b. **Nonatopic asthma** is characterized by chronic inflammation of the bronchi and bronchioles. The cause of the inflammation is not always obvious, but it may be initiated by viral infection and perpetuated by air pollutants. Adults are affected most often. Nonatopic asthma is often associated with chronic bronchitis (evidenced by coughing, even in between asthma attacks).
   c. **Occupational asthma** is an IgG-mediated response initiated by lung injury as a result of inhalation of fumes, dusts, or chemicals. This type of asthma, which primarily affects adults, is associated with chronic bronchitis and emphysema.

2. Pathologic findings in all types of asthma are uniform and include:
   a. **Inflammatory cell infiltrates** in the bronchial wall, with **prominent eosinophils**
   b. **Hyperplasia of the smooth muscle cells** and **bronchial glands** in the walls of the bronchi
   c. **Curschmann spirals** (spirals formed of shed epithelium) and **Charcot-Leyden crystals** (crystalloids derived from eosinophil granules) in the mucus that fills the bronchi **("mucous plugs")** or the sputum

 Status asthmaticus is sudden death owing to suffocation as a result of mucous plugging of bronchi.

B. **Chronic obstructive pulmonary disease (COPD)** includes two entities, emphysema and chronic bronchitis. Patients are categorized according to which entity predominates (Table 8-1).

1. **Emphysema.** Loss of the alveolar septa causes widening of the air spaces distal to the terminal bronchioles.
   a. **Centriacinar emphysema** is typically related to smoking and is characterized by inflammation and dilatation of the respiratory bronchioles. The walls of the respiratory bronchioles usually contain black carbon particles; the surrounding alveoli are relatively preserved.
   b. **Panacinar emphysema** is typically related to α_1-antitrypsin deficiency and is characterized by widening of the entire pulmonary acinus following destruc-

Table 8-1
Chronic Obstructive Pulmonary Disease (COPD)

	Predominantly Emphysema	Predominantly Chronic Bronchitis
Clinical appearance	"Pink puffer;" barrel-shaped, thin chest	"Blue bloater;" barrel-shaped, muscular chest
Age at onset	55–80 years	45–60 years
Symptoms		
Dyspnea	Mild, slowly progressive	Early onset, exacerbated during infection
Sputum production	Scant, mucoid	Copious, purulent
Weight loss	Prominent	Not evident
Chest auscultation	No abnormal sounds	Rhonchi ("noisy chest")
Radiologic findings	Hyperlucent lungs	Prominent bronchial tree and peribronchial fibrosis
Sputum bacteriology	Negative	Positive

tion of the alveolar walls by enzymes (e.g., elastase, protease). This type of emphysema is more prominent in the lower lobes.

2. **Chronic bronchitis** is clinically defined as a persistent, productive cough that lasts for at least 3 months, and occurs in 2 or more consecutive years. Bronchi are infiltrated with chronic inflammatory cells and the Reid index (i.e., the ratio of the thickness of the submucosal gland layer to that of the bronchial wall) is increased, owing to hypertrophy of the mucous-secreting glands.

IV. INTERSTITIAL LUNG DISEASES are classified functionally as **restrictive** because they restrict normal lung movements during respiration.

A. **Idiopathic pulmonary fibrosis** is a term used to refer to a group of restrictive lung diseases of unknown etiology. The most common is usual interstitial pneumonia (UIP).

1. On gross examination, the fibrotic lung contains numerous cysts (**"honeycomb lung"**).

2. Histologically, areas of fibrosis are interspersed among areas of focal inflammation and normal lung tissue.

> **NB**
>
> Similar pathologic changes may result from clinically identifiable causes (e.g., radiation, cytotoxic drugs, hypersensitivity reactions, pneumoconioses). Therefore, clinical data are essential for making the final diagnosis.

B. **Pneumoconioses** are caused by the inhalation of mineral contaminants.

1. **Coal workers' pneumoconiosis** (**"black lung disease"**) results from the inhalation of coal dust and encompasses several entities, including:
  a. Asymptomatic anthracosis
  b. Anthracosilicosis
  c. Progressive massive fibrosis (characterized by fibrosis, bronchiectasis, and pulmonary hypertension)
  d. Caplan syndrome (pneumoconiosis and rheumatoid lung disease)

2. Silicosis results from the inhalation of stone, sand, or flint dust containing **silica (silicon dioxide, SiO_2).** Silicosis results in small, fibrotic pulmonary nodules containing birefringent crystals.

> **NB**
>
> **Silicosis is associated with an increased predisposition to tuberculosis (silicotuberculosis).**

3. Asbestosis is caused by **asbestos fibers.** Asbestos bodies (visible by light microscopy as brown, beaded rods) cause pulmonary fibrosis, bronchogenic carcinoma, mesothelial plaques, and mesothelioma.

C. Hypersensitivity pneumonitis may be caused by a variety of organic dusts. The interstitial reaction (a type IV hypersensitivity reaction) results in the formation of loose granulomas and fibrosis. Examples include:

1. Byssinosis, a reaction to cotton or hemp fibers

2. Farmer's lung, a reaction to molds in hay dust

3. Silo-filler's lung, a reaction to nitrous oxides (found in corn-filled silos)

4. Bagassosis, a reaction to moldy sugar cane

D. Sarcoidosis is a systemic type IV hypersensitivity reaction to an unknown antigen that results in the formation of **noncaseating granulomas,** usually in the lungs and lymph nodes. The disorder is most common among young African-American women and has an unpredictable course. Two thirds of all patients recover spontaneously.

V. PULMONARY EMBOLISM is the obstruction of the pulmonary artery or its branches, usually by venous thromboemboli.

A. Large emboli occlude the **pulmonary trunk** or one of the **main pulmonary arteries** and are often **lethal.** An example is a **saddle embolus,** which lodges where the pulmonary artery bifurcates.

B. Medium-sized emboli tend to block the **segmental arteries** and may produce a wedge-shaped, red, hemorrhagic **pulmonary infarct,** especially in patients who have preexisting cardiopulmonary disease. (These patients are unable to establish collateral circulation, which would prevent the infarct.) Patients present with sudden pleural pain and subsequent hemoptysis.

C. Small emboli that are multiple and recurrent **("emboli showers")** tend to block the small branches of the pulmonary artery and over time may cause **pulmonary hypertension,** owing to a reduction in the diameter of the lumen of the blood vessels.

VI. PULMONARY INFECTIONS can be classified according to the etiology (e.g., bacterial, viral, or fungal), the location of the lesions (e.g., alveolar or interstitial), or the extent of lung involvement (e.g., diffuse, focal, unilateral, or bilateral).

A. Acute bacterial pneumonia

1. Bronchopneumonia (lobular pneumonia) is bacterial infection of the intrapulmonary bronchi, bronchioles, and adjacent alveoli. The exudate in these structures consists of polymorphonuclear neutrophils (PMNs), which accounts for the mucopurulent expectoration that characterizes this infection.

2. Lobar pneumonia, a diffuse alveolar infection involving an entire lobe or lung, is caused by *Streptococcus pneumoniae* in 90% of cases. This infection is most often seen in debilitated or terminally ill patients (e.g., elderly patients, alcoholic patients, cancer patients).

B. **Atypical (interstitial) pneumonia** is caused by **intracellular pathogens** such as **viruses** [e.g., adenovirus, paramyxovirus, cytomegalovirus (CMV)], *Mycoplasma pneumoniae,* and *Chlamydia pneumoniae,* which infect alveolar cells. The alveolar septa are usually edematous and contain an inflammatory **lymphocytic infiltrate.**

> **Because these pathogens attract mostly lymphocytes, PMNs are not present and there is no purulent expectoration—hence the term "atypical pneumonia."**

C. **Lung abscess.** A lung abscess is a localized area of liquefactive necrosis in the pulmonary parenchyma.

   1. *Staphylococcus aureus* and *Klebsiella pneumoniae* are most often isolated.

   2. Mechanisms of infection include aspiration of infective material from the upper respiratory or gastrointestinal tracts, pulmonary infarction by septic emboli, and bronchial obstruction by foreign bodies or tumors.

D. **Tuberculosis** is a granulomatous, chronic infection caused by *Mycobacterium tuberculosis*. The infection is most often limited to the lungs and bronchial lymph nodes, but it may spread to other organs via hematogenous dissemination.

   1. **Primary infection** is manifested by the **Ghon complex,** which consists of an intraparenchymal granulomatous lesion, usually located subpleurally in the midsection of the lungs, and hilar lymphadenopathy. In most cases, this infection resolves spontaneously.

   2. **Secondary infection** is reinfection, or, more often, reactivation of a latent but incompletely healed primary infection. The lesions of secondary tuberculosis are classically **apical.**
      a. **Cavitary tuberculosis** is extensive necrosis of the parenchymal lesion, leading to loss of the parenchyma and bleeding from severed vessels.
      b. **Miliary tuberculosis** is characterized by numerous minute nodules (i.e., 1- to 3-mm in diameter) resulting from the dissemination of M. *tuberculosis* through the lymphatic system or airways. Involvement may be limited to the lungs or extended to other organs.

E. **Fungal infections** are most common in debilitated or immunocompromised patients. The typical lesions of pulmonary fungal infections are **caseating granulomas.**

> **Necrotizing granulomas caused by fungi are clinically indistinguishable from those caused by *M. tuberculosis!* Special stains must be used to identify the pathogen in each case.**

   1. **Invasive candidiasis** and **invasive aspergillosis** are common in terminally ill patients and patients who are being treated with cytotoxic drugs.

   2. **Histoplasmosis, blastomycosis,** and **coccidioidosis** are prevalent in the Southwestern and Midwestern United States.

3. *Pneumocystis carinii* pneumonia (PCP) is an intraalveolar infection, typically seen in patients with AIDS. Unlike most other pulmonary fungal infections, PCP does not evoke an inflammatory response and is not characterized by a granulomatous reaction.

VII. PULMONARY NEOPLASMS. Lung tumors are the leading cause of cancer death in the United States. Approximately 90% of lung tumors are related to smoking tobacco.

A. General information

    1. **Incidence.** The incidence of lung cancer is second only to breast cancer (in women) and prostate carcinoma (in men).

    2. **Characteristics**
        a. Most lung tumors **are malignant.**
        b. Central tumors **are more common than peripheral (subpleural) ones.**
        c. Metastases to the lungs **are more common than primary lung tumors.** Metastases typically present as round ("cannonball") nodules.

B. Primary lung tumors (Table 8-2)

    1. **Squamous cell carcinomas** arise centrally from foci of squamous metaplasia in patients with chronic bronchitis caused by smoking.

    2. **Adenocarcinomas,** the most common form of lung cancer in nonsmokers, can occur in the hilus but are usually peripherally located and associated with scar tissue. Histologically, these tumors may be indistinguishable from metastatic adenocarcinomas.

    3. **Small cell lung carcinomas (oat cell carcinomas)** are composed of small cells that have neuroendocrine features (e.g., neuroendocrine granules on examination with an electron microscope, immunohistochemical reactivity with antibodies to chromogranin or synaptophysin). These rapidly growing tumors respond favorably to chemotherapy but are prone to early metastases; typically, they recur, causing death 18–20 months after diagnosis.

    4. **Undifferentiated large cell carcinomas** are composed of cells that do not show signs of differentiation. These tumors most likely evolve from either poorly differentiated adenocarcinomas of squamous cell carcinomas.

    5. **Carcinoid** is a low-grade malignant tumor (usually centrally located) composed of neuroendocrine cells. These tumors tend to invade and metastasize locally but are still associated with a 5-year survival rate of 90%.

    6. **Mesothelioma** is a malignant tumor of the pleura. Although mesothelioma does not metastasize distally, it is invariably lethal within 2 years.

Table 8-2
Primary Lung Tumors

Tumor	Approximate Incidence
Squamous cell carcinoma	35%
Adenocarcinoma	35%
Small cell lung carcinoma (oat cell)	20%
Undifferentiated large cell carcinoma	10%
Carcinoid	1%–2%
Mesothelioma	1%

Primary lung tumors most often metastasize to the local lymph nodes and mediastinum, the other lung, bone, the central nervous system (CNS), adrenal glands, and liver. To remember these sites, think **LOCAL:**
Lymph nodes and Lung
Osseous sites
CNS
Adrenal glands
Liver

C. Clinical features

1. Pulmonary signs and symptoms include a **productive, unremitting cough** with occasional hemoptysis; wheezing; dyspnea; chest pain; and **recurrent pulmonary infections.**

2. Systemic symptoms
   a. General systemic symptoms include **weight loss, weakness, and anorexia.**
   b. Signs associated with metastasis may include **pleural effusion, mediastinal compression syndromes, neurologic symptoms, pathologic fractures,** or **hepatomegaly.**
   c. Paraneoplastic syndromes
      (1) Small cell lung cancers (oat cell carcinomas) secrete polypeptide hormones and may cause **Cushing syndrome** or **syndrome of inappropriate antidiuretic hormone secretion (SIADH).**
      (2) **Squamous cell carcinomas** may secrete parathyroid hormone–related polypeptide (PTHrP), leading to **hypercalcemia.**
   d. **Carcinoid syndrome.** Patients with pulmonary (or gastrointestinal) carcinoids may develop carcinoid syndrome, which is characterized by facial flushing (due to vasomotor disturbances), diarrhea (due to intestinal hypermotility), or wheezing (due to bronchoconstriction).

9

Pathology of the Hematopoietic and Lymphoid Systems

I. INTRODUCTION. The clinical manifestations of diseases of the hematopoietic and lymphoid systems are related to either a deficiency or an excess of blood or lymphoid cells.

A. Blood or lymphoid cell deficiency

1. **Anemia** is present when the red blood cell (RBC) count is less than 4.5×10^{12} cells/L (4.1×10^{12} cells/L in women) or the hemoglobin level is less than 13.5 g/dl (11.5 g/dl in women).

> **The normal RBC count of 5×10^{12} cells/L is known in common parlance as 5 million RBCs per microliter!**

   a. **Clinical features** (e.g., pallor, shortness of breath, easy fatigability, somnolence) result from an inadequate supply of oxygen to the organs and tissues.

   b. **Morphologic classification** is based on microscopic examination of peripheral blood smears (Figure 9-1).

   (1) **Normocytic-normochromic.** The RBCs are of normal size and color.

   (2) **Microcytic-hypochromic.** The RBCs are small and contain less hemoglobin than normal. The mean corpuscular volume (MCV) is 60–70 femtoliters per RBC.

   (3) **Macrocytic-hyperchromic.** The RBCs are large (MCV $\geq$ 100 fl/RBC) and lack central pallor.

   c. **Mechanisms of anemia** include:

   (1) Decreased RBC production

   (2) Increased RBC destruction

   (3) Blood loss (i.e., acute or chronic hemorrhage)

2. **Leukopenia,** a reduction in the number of white blood cells (WBCs), is manifested as a reduced resistance to infection.

3. **Thrombocytopenia,** a reduction in the number of platelets, results in a bleeding tendency.

B. Blood or lymphoid cell excess. An excess of circulating blood cells is usually associated with hypercellularity of the bone marrow or lymphoid organs and the spleen. It may be **reactive** (e.g., secondary polycythemia in a patient who lives at a high altitude; leukocytosis in infection) or **neoplastic** (e.g., leukemia).

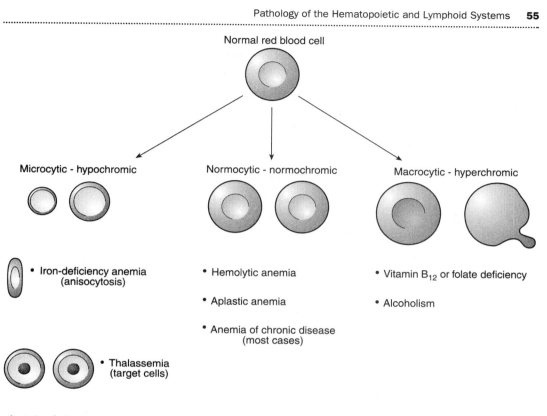

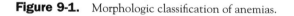

Figure 9-1.   Morphologic classification of anemias.

1. Polycythemia (erythrocytosis) is an increase in the number of circulating RBCs. The blood is viscous and the skin and mucosae appear dark red.

2. Leukocytosis (i.e., an excess of mature leukocytes in the blood) does not, in and of itself, cause symptoms.

> **NB**
>
> **A leukemoid reaction (i.e., an exaggerated form of leukocytosis) must be distinguished from leukemia (i.e., a neoplastic disease). The normal leukocytes of a leukemoid reaction express alkaline phosphatase (AP), which is not present in the abnormal leukocytes of leukemia.**

3. Thrombocytosis, an increase in the number of circulating platelets, is marked by increased coagulability of the blood. Thrombocytosis may be reactive, but is most often related to neoplastic diseases (e.g., myeloproliferative syndromes).

II. ANEMIAS CAUSED BY DECREASED RED BLOOD CELL (RBC) PRODUCTION.
Causes of impaired RBC production include bone marrow failure and inadequate supplies of the components necessary for forming RBCs (e.g., iron, folic acid, vitamin B_{12}).

A. Aplastic anemia. Fat cells replace hematopoietic cells in the bone marrow, resulting in anemia, leukopenia, and thrombocytopenia.

  1. Cause. In most cases, the cause is not known, but aplastic anemia may be related to drug therapy, toxins, or radiation.

  2. Therapy. Stem cell populations can be replenished by bone marrow transplantation, but in spite of therapy, many patients die, usually as a result of infection.

B. Iron-deficiency anemia is the most common cause of anemia.

  1. Causes. A negative iron balance may result from:
   a. Inadequate iron intake or absorption (e.g., as a result of dietary deficiency, achlorhydria, or celiac disease)
   b. Excessive iron loss (e.g., as a result of menstruation or chronic gastrointestinal bleeding)
   c. Increased iron demand (e.g., during pregnancy, lactation, or infancy)

  2. Pathologic findings include:
   a. A **microcytic–hypochromic anemia** with **anisocytosis** (i.e., cigar- or pencil-shaped cells)
   b. Low bone marrow iron stores
   c. Low serum iron and **ferritin levels**
   d. Low transferrin saturation
   e. High total iron binding capacity (TIBC)

C. Vitamin B_{12} and folate deficiencies adversely affect DNA synthesis in hematopoietic cells and hinder the maturation of bone marrow precursors of blood cells. Anemia caused by vitamin B_{12} deficiency is called **pernicious anemia.**

  1. Causes. These nutritional deficiencies may result from:
   a. Malabsorption of vitamin B_{12} (e.g., as may occur in type A gastritis, Crohn disease, or parasitic infection of the small intestine)
   b. Inadequate intake of folic acid (e.g., as a result of malnutrition or alcoholism)
   c. Increased demand for folic acid (e.g., as occurs during pregnancy)
   d. Drug therapy with agents that interfere with absorption or act as folate antagonists, such as methotrexate

  2. Pathologic findings
   a. On peripheral blood smears, the **RBCs** are **macrocytic** and often **hyperchromic. Neutrophils** are **hypersegmented.**
   b. The bone marrow contains numerous **megaloblasts** (i.e., immature RBC precursors that are much larger than normoblasts).
   c. The **platelet count** is **low.**
   d. The serum **vitamin B_{12}** or **folate levels are low.**

D. Thalassemia is a term used to refer to a group of anemias caused by defective synthesis of hemoglobin A (HbA), a tetramer composed of two α and two β chains ($\alpha_2\beta_2$).

  1. Pathogenesis. Two factors contribute to the anemia seen in thalassemia:
   a. The overall concentration of normal hemoglobin A (HbA-$\alpha_2\beta_2$) is reduced.
   b. An abnormal ratio of α chains to β chains results in intracellular deposits, producing characteristic **target cells,** which are prone to hemolysis.

  2. Types of thalassemia

    a. β-Thalassemia, the most common form of thalassemia, is related to mutation of one or both of the genes that code for β globin.

        (1) **Thalassemia major (Cooley anemia).** Patients homozygous for the mutated β globin gene develop hemolysis, splenomegaly, bone marrow hyperplasia, and bone deformities.

        (2) **Thalassemia minor** is a mild anemia that occurs in heterozygous patients.

    b. α-Thalassemia is related to the deletion of one or more of the four α globin genes; clinical features may be severe or mild, depending on the number of deleted genes.

III. ANEMIAS CAUSED BY INCREASED RED BLOOD CELL (RBC) DESTRUCTION.

Hemolysis may be **acute** (as in transfusion reactions) or **chronic** (as in hemolytic anemia). It may be **intravascular** (i.e., occurring within the blood vessel) or **extravascular** (i.e., occurring within the phagocytic cells of the spleen and liver).

A. Classification of hemolytic anemias

    1. **Intracorpuscular.** Hemolysis results from intrinsic RBC abnormalities, such as those affecting structural proteins (e.g., spectrin, ankyrin), the globin portion of hemoglobin, or RBC enzymes [e.g., glucose-6-phosphate dehydrogenase (G6PD)].

        a. **Hereditary spherocytosis** is an autosomal dominant condition, most often related to spectrin deficiency. RBCs lacking spectrin are removed by the spleen. Splenectomy is curative.

        b. **Sickle cell anemia** is a hemoglobinopathy affecting 8% of African-Americans. A mutation in the gene coding for the β globin chain results in the formation of sickle hemoglobin (hemoglobin S, HbS), which attains a sickle shape under hypoxic conditions. Clinical features of sickle cell disease (Figure 9-2) depend on the amount of HbS, which varies from 40% in heterozygotes to 100% in homozygotes.

    2. **Extracorpuscular.** Factors extrinsic to the RBC result in hemolysis.

        a. **Mechanical hemolysis** occurs inside the blood vessels or heart chambers. Causes include prostheses (e.g., heart valves) and microangiopathic diseases [e.g., disseminated intravascular coagulation (DIC)].

        b. **Autoimmune hemolytic anemia**

            (1) The **warm antibody type,** the most common form of autoimmune hemolytic anemia, is IgG-mediated. The warm antibody type is a feature of systemic lupus erythematosus (SLE) and related autoimmune diseases, and of drug-related hypersensitivity reactions.

            (2) The **cold antibody type** is IgM-mediated and may occur acutely (e.g., following infectious mononucleosis) or chronically (e.g., in patients with lymphoma).

B. **Pathologic findings** in hemolytic anemia include compensatory **bone marrow hyperplasia, reticulocytosis,** and **hemosiderin deposits** (as a result of iron storage).

C. **Clinical features** of hemolytic anemias include **jaundice** (owing to unconjugated hyperbilirubinemia), **splenomegaly,** and **hepatomegaly.**

IV. BLEEDING DISORDERS,

which may be either congenital or acquired, result from abnormalities of the vessel wall, platelets, or clotting factors. The classification of bleeding disorders is given in Table 9-1.

A. **Thrombocytopenia** is defined as a platelet count of less than 100,000 cells/μl. Spontaneous bleeding occurs only if the platelet count is less than 20,000 cells/μl. Causes of thrombocytopenia include:

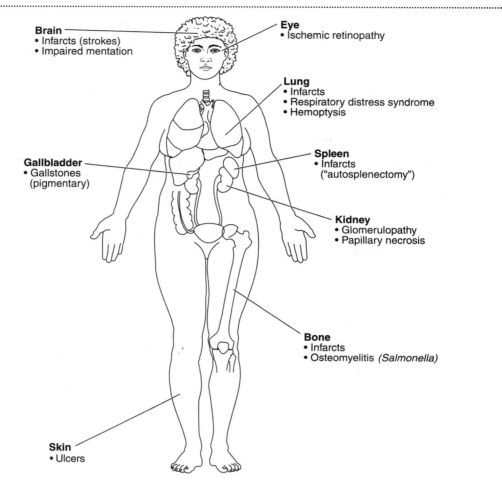

Brain
• Infarcts (strokes)
• Impaired mentation

Eye
• Ischemic retinopathy

Lung
• Infarcts
• Respiratory distress syndrome
• Hemoptysis

Gallbladder
• Gallstones
  (pigmentary)

Spleen
• Infarcts
  ("autosplenectomy")

Kidney
• Glomerulopathy
• Papillary necrosis

Bone
• Infarcts
• Osteomyelitis *(Salmonella)*

Skin
• Ulcers

Figure 9-2. Clinical features of sickle cell disease result from intra- and extravascular hemolysis of sickled cells, leading to anemia, and occlusion of the microvascular by sickled cells, leading to ischemia. Although hemoglobin S (HbS) is the predominant hemoglobinopathy in sickle cell disease, other abnormal hemoglobins [e.g., hemoglobin C (HbC)] may aggravate symptoms.

    1. Decreased platelet production as a result of bone marrow failure

    2. Increased platelet removal as a result of hypersplenism

    3. Decreased platelet survival (e.g., as a result of immune-mediated disorders or DIC)

    4. Cytotoxic drug therapy

    5. Infection (e.g., AIDS)

B. Idiopathic thrombocytopenic purpura (ITP) is an autoimmune disorder caused by antibodies to platelets, megakaryocytes, or both. Opsonized platelets are removed by the spleen and liver. Two clinical forms are recognized:

    1. Acute ITP is a self-limited disease, usually related to an infection, that affects children.

Table 9-1
Classification of Bleeding Disorders

Classification	Examples	Laboratory Findings
Disorders of primary hemostasis	Vascular disorders (e.g., hyper-sensitivity vasculitis), thrombocytopenia, thrombasthenia	Prolonged bleeding time
Disorders of secondary hemostasis	Clotting factor deficiencies (e.g., vitamin K deficiency, hemophilia)	Prolonged aPTT
Disorders of primary and secondary hemostasis	von Willebrand disease, thrombo-cytopenic microangiopathies (e.g., DIC, ITP, TTP)	Prolonged bleeding time and aPTT; normal or prolonged PT

aPTT = activated partial thromboplastin time; DIC = disseminated intravascular coagulation; ITP = idiopathic thrombocytopenic purpura; PT = prothrombin time; TTP = thrombotic thrombocytopenic purpura.

2. Chronic ITP, a disorder that affects women between the ages of 20 and 40 years, is mediated by antibodies to platelet surface antigens (i.e., IIb/IIIa and Ib).

C. Thrombotic microangiopathic purpura is a term used to describe several conditions characterized by the formation of platelet–fibrin thrombi in small blood vessels, leading to depletion of clotting factors (i.e., consumption coagulopathy).

1. Thrombotic thrombocytopenic purpura (TTP) typically affects women. Clinical features include renal failure, fever, neurologic symptoms, hemolytic anemia, and thrombocytopenia.

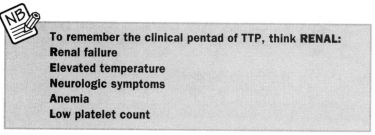

To remember the clinical pentad of TTP, think **RENAL:**
Renal failure
Elevated temperature
Neurologic symptoms
Anemia
Low platelet count

2. Hemolytic–uremic syndrome (HUS) is similar to TTP, but it occurs in children and does not present with neurologic symptoms. It is often caused by infection with enterotoxigenic *Escherichia coli.*

3. DIC is a consumption coagulopathy that often accompanies disorders associated with the activation of thrombin (e.g., shock, sepsis, terminal cancer). Depletion of fibrin and other coagulation factors leads to hemorrhage, which may be difficult to stop. Fibrin split products appear in the urine owing to plasmin-mediated fibrinolysis.

D. Clotting factor deficiencies may be acquired (e.g., liver disease, vitamin K deficiency, DIC) or congenital (e.g., hemophilia, von Willebrand disease).

1. Hemophilia A and B are X-linked disorders caused by mutations of the genes that code for factors VIII and IX, respectively.
   a. Clinical features include spontaneous or post-traumatic bleeding, hematoma

formation in soft tissue and muscle, and hemarthrosis leading to joint deformity.

    b. **Laboratory findings.** Patients have a normal bleeding time and platelet count, but the activated partial thromboplastin time (aPTT) is prolonged.

2. **von Willebrand disease** is characterized by a deficiency of von Willebrand factor (vWF), a substance that both stabilizes factor VIII and plays a role in the adhesion of platelets to the endothelium. The most common hereditary bleeding disorder, von Willebrand disease is usually inherited as an autosomal dominant disorder, although autosomal recessive variants have been identified.

    a. **Clinical features** vary, but may include prolonged bleeding during menstruation or following a minor wound, or spontaneous bleeding from the gums and other sites.

    b. **Laboratory findings.** Because vWF mediates adhesion of platelets and also serves as a carrier for factor VIII, both the bleeding time and the aPTT are prolonged.

V. BONE MARROW NEOPLASIA

A. Introduction

    1. **Mechanisms of disease in bone marrow neoplasia**

        a. Malignant cells (blasts) overpopulate the bone marrow and replace the normal cells, causing bone destruction (as in multiple myeloma) or blood or lymphoid cell deficiencies.

        b. Malignant cells and their descendants may appear in the circulating blood (as in leukemia), in extramedullary sites, such as the spleen and liver (resulting in hepatosplenomegaly), and in lymph nodes (resulting in lymphadenopathy).

        c. Bone marrow malignancy may be accompanied by myelofibrosis.

    Myelofibrosis, seen on bone marrow biopsy and typically associated with anemia, may be the first sign of neoplasia!

    2. **Types of bone marrow neoplasia.** Malignant transformation of hematopoietic and lymphoid cell precursors may occur at any stage of their development. Malignant cells are classified as myeloid, lymphoid, or plasmacytic. The biology of the malignant stem cell determines the clinical presentation of the disease, leading to four major groups of diseases:

        a. **Myeloproliferative disorders,** which are characterized by the malignant transformation of developmentally pluripotent myeloid stem cells and their cell lineage–restricted descendants

        b. **Myelodysplastic syndromes,** which are characterized by ineffective hematopoiesis and pancytopenia

        c. **Leukemias,** which are characterized by the appearance of neoplastic WBCs in the circulation ("white blood")

        d. **Plasma cell disorders,** which result from the monoclonal proliferation of neoplastic plasma cells and plasmacytoid lymphocytes, usually in the bone marrow

B. **Myeloproliferative disorders** include **polycythemia rubra vera** (caused by the proliferation of RBC precursors), **essential thrombocytopenia** (caused by the proliferation of platelet precursors), **chronic myelocytic leukemia** (CML; caused by the proliferation of neutrophil precursors), and **myelofibrosis** (caused by the proliferation of fibroblasts). These four clinical entities are interrelated and may transform, either one into another or into acute myeloblastic leukemia (AML). Clinical features common to all of the myeloproliferative disorders include:

1. Peak incidence in the 40- to 70-year age group

2. Bone marrow hypercellularity (except in myelofibrosis, which is dominated by fibrosis)

3. Splenomegaly as a result of extramedullary hematopoiesis (especially in myelofibrosis)

4. Peripheral blood abnormalities (e.g., erythrocytosis, thrombocytosis, leukemia) and hyperviscosity of the blood (especially in polycythemia rubra vera)

> **In order to distinguish polycythemia rubra vera from secondary polycythemia, look at the serum erythropoietin level—it is elevated in secondary polycythemia, but normal in polycythemia rubra vera because the neoplastic proliferation of erythroid cells occurs independently of erythropoietin.**

C. Leukemias. Two major groups of leukemias are recognized: **myeloid (granulocytic)** and **lymphoid.**

1. Causes. The cause of leukemia is not known, although some predisposing factors have been identified. In some cases, a myelodysplastic syndrome precedes the onset of leukemia.

a. Genetic factors may play a role, as evidenced by the higher incidence of leukemia in patients with chromosomal syndromes (e.g., Down syndrome, Bloom syndrome, Fanconi syndrome).

b. Ionizing radiation. Atomic bomb survivors and patients who have undergone radiation therapy may develop leukemia.

c. Alkylating agents used in cancer therapy may cause leukemia.

d. Viruses. Human T-cell lymphotropic virus-1 (HTLV-1) is an RNA oncogenic virus that causes human T-cell leukemia.

e. Endogenous oncogenes play a role and are associated with chromosomal breaks, translocations, or deletions. Best known is the **Philadelphia chromosome,** associated with the development of **CML.** The Philadelphia chromosome is formed by the translocation of fragments of chromosomes 9 and 22 and leads to the formation of a hybrid oncogene, *bcr-c-abl.*

2. Types of leukemias (Table 9-2)

a. Acute lymphoblastic leukemia (ALL) accounts for 30% of all leukemias and is the most common leukemia in children younger than 5 years.

b. Acute myelogenous leukemia (AML) accounts for 80% of acute leukemias in adults. AML may start *de novo,* or it may be the end-stage of CML and myelofibrosis.

c. Chronic lymphocytic leukemia (CLL) has a long, slow course (7–9 years) and does not respond to chemotherapy. CLL is closely related to small cell lymphocytic lymphoma; therefore, lymphadenopathy is a common feature.

d. Chronic myelocytic leukemia (CML) has a clinical course that lasts 2–3 years, usually terminating in a fatal blast crisis. Symptoms (e.g., anemia, bleeding, infection) are related to the loss of normal bone marrow cells.

Table 9-2
Leukemias

Type	Peak Incidence	Bone Marrow and Peripheral Blood Findings	Clinical-Pathological Classification	Prognosis
Acute lymphocytic leukemia (ALL)	Childhood	Bone marrow contains > 30% lymphoblasts	L_1: Small lymphoblastic L_2: Large lymphoblastic L_3: Undifferentiated	Very good in children; less favorable in adults
Acute myelogenous leukemia (AML)	Adulthood	Bone marrow contains > 30% myeloblasts	French-American-British classification (M_1–M_7)	Poor; most patients relapse following chemo-therapy and die within 5 years
Chronic lymphocytic leukemia (CLL)	Men older than 60 years	Bone marrow contains > 40% lymphoid cells; peripheral blood contains > 15,000 × 10^6 WBCs/L; neoplastic cells resemble B lympho-cytes and express the *bcl*-2 oncogene	. . .	Variable; many patients live for several years after diagnosis and die from unrelated causes
Chronic myelocytic leukemia (CML)	Age 60 years	Bone marrow is hyper-cellular and contains blasts as well as more mature cells; peripheral blood contains 20,000–50,000 × 10^6 WBCs/L, including myeloid precursors (e.g., myeloblasts, myelo-cytes) and more mature PMNs; during blast crisis, WBC count increases to >100,000 × 10^6/L	. . .	Poor; remission can be induced by chemo-therapy, but the disease recurs and is almost always fatal

PMNs = polymorphonuclear neutrophils; WBCs= white blood cells.

D. Plasma cell disorders

   1. Overview

      a. Types of plasma cell disorders

         (1) Multiple myeloma

         (2) Waldenström macroglobulinemia

         (3) Monoclonal gammopathy of unknown significance (MGUS)

         (4) Solitary plasmacytoma

      b. Clinical features of plasma cell disorders

         (1) They occur in patients older than 45 years.

         (2) The **neoplastic plasma cells secrete a monoclonal immunoglobulin,** which can be recognized by serum electrophoresis.

(3) The light chain of the immunoglobulin may form amyloid, which is deposited in the kidneys, blood vessels, and other organs **(amyloidosis).**

2. Multiple myeloma is a neoplasm of mature plasma cells. Patients do not respond to chemotherapy and usually die within 3 years of the onset of disease. Kidney damage is the most common cause of death (60% of patients). Other causes of death include infection (20% of patients), systemic amyloidosis (10% of patients), anemia or hyperviscosity of the blood, and metabolic disorders.

a. The neoplastic cells secrete a monoclonal immunoglobulin called **M component.** M component is most often an IgG (60% of patients). IgA (20% of cases) and either IgD, IgE, or the light or heavy chain of an immunoglobulin (20% of cases) are less common. Normal immunoglobulins are suppressed, increasing the patient's susceptibility to infections.

b. Multiple bone lesions composed of neoplastic plasma cells appear as **punched-out defects** on radiographs. Hypercalcemia from the lytic bone lesions causes calciuria, polyuria, and metastatic calcification.

c. Excess immunoglobulin light chains may be deposited in tissues (most often in the kidneys and blood vessels), where they form **amyloid fibers,** or secreted in the urine as **Bence Jones protein.**

d. Immunoglobulins form obstructive casts in the renal tubules (**"myeloma kidney"**).

3. Waldenström macroglobulinemia. The neoplastic cells of Waldenström macroglobulinemia, called **plasmacytoid lymphocytes,** have features of both B lymphocytes and plasma cells and secrete **immunoglobulin M (IgM, macroglobulin).** IgM causes hyperviscosity of the blood, leading to **retinal** and **cerebral ischemia** as a result of blockage of the microvasculature.

4. MGUS is a laboratory diagnosis most often made in asymptomatic elderly patients. The disorder is innocuous in most cases, but 20% of patients ultimately develop plasma cell neoplasia.

VI. LYMPHOMAS are neoplasms of lymphoid cells. Two major groups are recognized: **non-Hodgkin lymphoma** (70% of cases) and **Hodgkin disease** (30% of cases).

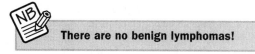

There are no benign lymphomas!

A. Causes. The cause of lymphoma is unknown, but some possible predisposing factors have been identified:

1. Oncogenes. Lymphomas are closely related to leukemias and could be caused by the same oncogenes (e.g., *bcl-2* is present in the neoplastic cells of CLL, and in well-differentiated B cell lymphoma cells).

2. Radiation. The incidence of lymphoma is increased in patients who have been exposed to radiation.

3. Environmental factors may play a pathogenetic role. For example, Burkitt lymphoma, predominant in sub-Saharan Africa, is related to Epstein-Barr virus (EBV) infection.

4. Immunodeficiency states (congenital and acquired) are associated with an increased incidence of lymphomas, some of which occur in unusual places (e.g., the CNS).

B. Non-Hodgkin lymphomas are a heterogeneous group of neoplasms originating from B and T lymphocytes and their precursors.

1. **Origin and areas of involvement.** Most (85%) of non-Hodgkin lymphomas are of B-cell origin and involve the lymph nodes, bone marrow, spleen, or extranodal lymphoid tissue.

   a. Approximately two thirds of cases originate in the lymph nodes. The remaining third are extranodal [e.g., gastrointestinal lymphomas originating from mucosa-associated lymphoid tissue (MALT)].

   b. Multiple lymph nodes at a distance from one another are usually involved, owing to the migratory nature of lymphoid cells.

2. **Classification schemes**

   a. The **National Institutes of Health (NIH) Working Classification** scheme classifies lymphomas clinically as **high-grade, low-grade,** or **intermediate.** As a rule, low-grade lymphomas have an indolent course, whereas high-grade lymphomas respond to chemotherapy but recur and are lethal.

   b. The **Revised European American Lymphoma (REAL)** classification scheme is based on the immunophenotyping of tumor cells. Four general categories are recognized:

      (1) **Precursor B-cell neoplasms** comprise several entities, such as **acute lymphoblastic lymphoma** of infancy and childhood, and **high-grade lymphoblastic lymphoma** of adulthood. These lymphomas respond well to chemotherapy but often recur, especially in adults. Acute lymphoblastic lymphoma in children is often curable.

      (2) **Precursor T-cell neoplasms** may respond to chemotherapy, but usually less favorably than precursor B-cell neoplasms.

      (3) **Peripheral B-cell neoplasms** account for most cases of non-Hodgkin lymphomas in adults. This group comprises more than 20 entities, which vary in their clinical course.

         (a) **Small cell lymphocytic lymphoma** is the lymphoma equivalent of CLL. Like CLL, small cell lymphocytic lymphoma has a protracted course (7–9 years) and is incurable.

         (b) **Follicular lymphoma** also has a protracted course.

         (c) **Mantle cell lymphoma** and **diffuse large B-cell lymphoma** are lethal 2–3 years after diagnosis, despite an initial response to chemotherapy.

         (d) **Hairy cell leukemia** is a low-grade lymphoma associated with splenomegaly. Leukemia results from "spillover" of hairy lymphocytes into the peripheral blood.

         (e) **Burkitt lymphoma,** which affects children and young adults, has a poor prognosis.

      (4) **Peripheral T-cell** and **natural killer (NK) cell neoplasms.** This very heterogeneous group of neoplasms includes low-grade, intermediate, and high grade neoplasms.

         (a) **Mycosis fungoides** is a dermatotropic low-grade lymphoma related to **Sézary syndrome,** a form of low-grade T-cell leukemia.

         (b) **Peripheral T-cell lymphoma, unspecified** is the largest group of neoplasms in this category. These tumors usually respond initially to chemotherapy but invariably kill the patient 1–2 years after diagnosis.

C. Hodgkin disease comprises several neoplastic lymph node disorders that resemble lymphoma.

1. **Areas of involvement.** The neoplastic process involves contiguous lymph nodes (usually of the neck and mediastinum), suggesting local spreading. The Waldeyer ring of the nasopharynx and extranodal tissues are rarely involved.

2. **Pathologic findings**
   a. The affected lymph nodes show an inflammatory response to tumor cells and contain **infiltrates of other cells,** such as plasma cells and eosinophils.
   b. **Reed-Sternberg cells** (i.e., large, binucleated cells that look like **owl eyes**) are the basis of pathologic diagnosis. These cells are surrounded by other cells that allow pathologists to recognize **four histologic types** of Hodgkin disease:
      (1) Nodular sclerosis (the most common form)
      (2) Lymphocyte predominance
      (3) Lymphocyte depletion
      (4) Mixed cellularity

3. **Clinical features.** Some patients with Hodgkin disease have **"B symptoms"** characteristic of inflammatory disease (e.g., **fever, sweating, generalized malaise**).

> **Patients with "B symptoms" have a worse prognosis than those who do not have these symptoms.**

4. **Prognosis** depends primarily on the stage of disease, and to a lesser extent on histologic type. Generally, the response to chemotherapy is excellent, and 75% of patients survive for at least 5 years. When relapse does occur, it can be cured in 50% of cases.

10

Pathology of the Oral Cavity and Gastrointestinal Tract

I. DEVELOPMENTAL DISORDERS

A. **Cleft lip** and **cleft palate** are multifactorial disorders that often accompany each other and are more common in boys.

B. **Esophageal atresia** (i.e., failure of the lumen to develop) is usually accompanied by **tracheoesophageal fistula.** These are the most common esophageal developmental disorders.

C. **Hypertrophic pyloric stenosis** is caused by hypertrophy of the smooth muscle that surrounds the pylorus. The disorder is most common in boys. Patients present with projectile vomiting.

D. **Meckel diverticulum** occurs when the omphalomesenteric duct fails to involute, resulting in a blind pouch that protrudes from the small intestine.

> **Inflammation of a Meckel diverticulum presents as "left-sided appendicitis."**

E. **Hirschsprung disease (congenital megacolon)** is progressive dilatation of the segment of colon proximal to an aganglionic segment of the rectum.

II. INFLAMMATORY DISORDERS

A. **Stomatitis** is inflammation of the oral mucosa.

    1. **Aphthous stomatitis,** characterized by small, painful, shallow ulcers, is caused by viral infection.

    2. **Oral candidiasis (thrush)** is seen in infants and debilitated patients. The characteristic white plaques can be scraped away to reveal an inflammatory base.

    3. **Hairy leukoplakia,** characterized by white mucosal papules and caused by human papillomavirus (HPV) infection, is seen in HIV-positive patients.

B. **Sialadenitis** is inflammation of the salivary glands. Causes include:

    1. **Viral infection** (e.g., mumps)

2. Bacterial infection, which is often preceded by **sialolithiasis** (i.e., partial obstruction of the salivary duct by concrements)

3. Autoimmune disorders, such as **Sjögren syndrome**

C. **Esophagitis.** Causes include the following.

1. Chemical irritation may result from endogenous substances (e.g., gastric juices in **reflux esophagitis)** or exogenous substances (e.g., **strong acid** or **alkali,** like lye).

2. Viral infection. Esophagitis caused by viral infection occurs most often in immunosuppressed patients. Common etiologic agents include **herpes simplex virus (HSV)** and **cytomegalovirus (CMV).**

3. Fungal infection leading to esophagitis is most common in debilitated patients and patients with diabetes.

> **The esophagus is covered with squamous epithelium, which is resistant to bacterial infection!**

D. Gastritis

1. Acute erosive gastritis is caused by the overuse of nonsteroidal anti-inflammatory drugs (NSAIDs), such as aspirin, and alcohol.

2. Chronic gastritis
  a. Type A gastritis is caused by **autoantibodies** against parietal cells, resulting in destruction of the glands that secrete hydrochloric acid and intrinsic factor. The lack of intrinsic factor hinders absorption of vitamin B_{12}, leading to **pernicious anemia.**
  b. Type B gastritis is caused by *Helicobacter pylori* infection.

3. Hypertrophic gastritis includes several conditions, such as **Ménétrier disease,** which is idiopathic, and **hypergastrinemia,** which is caused by endocrine tumors in patients with Zollinger-Ellison syndrome.

E. **Peptic ulcer disease** is characterized by mucosal defects and deeper ulcerations in the stomach or duodenum. Causes include hyperacidity and *H. pylori* infection.

F. **Enteritis** is inflammation of the small intestine associated with diarrhea, malabsorption, or both.

1. Infectious causes
  a. Viruses (e.g., **rotavirus, Norwalk virus),** most common in children
  b. Bacteria
    (1) *Escherichia coli* (food-borne)
    (2) *Vibrio cholerae* (water-borne)
    (3) *Staphylococcus aureus,* which secretes a preformed toxin and causes "food poisoning"
    (4) *Mycobacterium avium-intracellulare* **(MAI),** which can cause enteritis in patients with AIDS
    (5)*Tropheryma whippelii,* the intracellular bacterium responsible for Whipple disease (a malabsorption syndrome)
  c. Parasites (e.g., *Giardia lamblia*)

2. Celiac sprue. Gluten intolerance leads to atrophy of the intestinal villi and, consequently, malabsorption.

    G. Appendicitis. Mixed bacterial infection (following luminal obstruction by fecaliths, parasites, or enlarged lymphoid follicles) leads to inflammation of the appendix.

    H. Colitis

        1. Infectious colitis. Forms include **shigellosis, salmonellosis, amebiasis,** and **pseudomembranous colitis** (caused by *Clostridium difficile*).

        2. Inflammatory bowel disease (IBD) comprises two closely related but distinct diseases of unknown etiology: **Crohn disease** and **ulcerative colitis** (Table 10-1).

    I. Gay bowel syndrome (infectious proctitis) is a sexually transmitted disease seen most often in male homosexuals with HIV infection. Gay bowel syndrome may be caused by viruses (HSV, CMV, HPV), bacteria, or fungi.

III. CIRCULATORY DISORDERS

    A. Esophageal varices are a complication of portal hypertension and are typically seen in patients with cirrhosis.

    B. Stress-related injury to the gastric mucosa, in the form of **erosions** and **ulcers,** can occur following shock, massive burns **("Curling ulcers"),** sepsis, and intracranial trauma **("Cushing ulcers").** Ischemia of the gastric mucosa (due to hypotension) plays a significant role in causing these lesions.

    C. Intestinal angiodysplasia is characterized by submucosal intestinal varicosities. These varicosities are prone to rupture, causing minute but prolonged blood loss and, subsequently, anemia.

    D. Ischemic colitis is characterized by nonhealing ischemic ulcerations of the colonic mucosa owing to atherosclerosis of the mesenteric vessels.

    E. Mesenteric thrombosis causes hemorrhagic infarcts of the intestines.

        1. Arterial thrombosis is most often seen in patients with atherosclerosis of the superior mesenteric artery.

        2. Venous thrombosis is most often seen in patients with hypercoagulable states, cancer, or cirrhosis, or following abdominal surgery.

    F. Hemorrhoids are varicosities of the anal and perianal submucosal venous plexuses. The dilated veins are prone to thrombosis or painful prolapse through the anus.

Table 10-1
Comparison of Crohn Disease and Ulcerative Colitis

	Ulcerative colitis	**Crohn disease**
Affected portion of the bowel	Rectum, colon	Ileum, colon
Distribution	Continuous	Patchy ("skip lesions")
Gross appearance	Broad, shallow ulcers	Deep fissures
	Pseudopolyps	"Cobblestone mucosa"
	Dilatations	Strictures
Microscopic findings	Crypt abscesses	Crypt abscesses
	Inflammation (limited to the mucosa)	Inflammation (transmural)
	No granulomas	Granulomas found in 50% of patients
	No fibrosis	Fibrosis
Complications	Megacolon	Fistulae, adhesions
	Carcinoma (++)	Carcinoma (+/−)

IV. GASTROINTESTINAL TRACT OBSTRUCTIONS AND DILATATIONS

A. **Obstructions** (Figure 10-1)

    1. **Intussusception** is obstruction caused by invagination of one segment of the intestine into another.

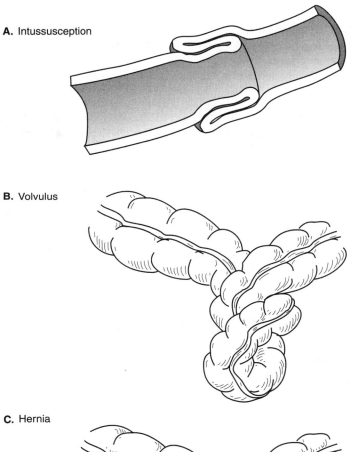

A. Intussusception

B. Volvulus

C. Hernia

Figure 10-1.   Intestinal obstructions.

2. Volvulus is the twisting of the bowel and its mesenteric root, resulting in intestinal obstruction and ischemic necrosis of the twisted intestinal loops.

3. Herniation is protrusion of the intestinal contents through a hole in the abdominal wall. Hernias are most often inguinal, but may be femoral or diaphragmatic. Only incarcerated, inflamed, or fibrotic hernias cause intestinal obstruction.

Paralytic ileus is functional obstruction of the small intestine resulting from loss of peristalsis due to trauma, peritonitis, sepsis, surgery, or shock.

Constipation (i.e., the inability to pass stools) may mimic intestinal obstruction but it is most often of functional origin and has no underlying pathology.

B. Dilatations

1. Diverticula are localized dilatations of the lumen caused by defects in the intestinal wall.

  a. Esophageal diverticula

   (1) Zenker diverticulum (upper esophagus)

   (2) Traction diverticulum (midportion)

  b. Colonic diverticulosis is a condition seen most often in elderly patients and characterized by **multiple colonic diverticula,** usually located in the sigmoid colon.

V. GASTROINTESTINAL NEOPLASMS

A. Oral cavity tumors. Squamous cell carcinoma may be *in situ* or invasive. Clinically, it may present as leukoplakia or erythroplakia, ulcers, or nodules.

B. Salivary gland tumors. Eighty percent of salivary gland tumors are benign.

1. Pleomorphic adenomas are usually found in the parotid gland. These tumors are usually benign but may recur and, in 3%–5% of cases, may undergo malignant transformation.

2. Mucoepidermoid carcinoma is the most common type of salivary gland carcinoma.

3. Cystic adenolymphoma (Warthin tumor) is a rare benign tumor occurring almost exclusively in the parotid gland.

C. Esophageal tumors. Most esophageal tumors are malignant.

1. Squamous cell carcinoma is most often seen in the upper two thirds of the esophagus.

2. Adenocarcinomas are thought to originate from dysplastic epithelium in patients with **Barrett esophagus,** a complication of long-standing gastroesophageal reflux that affects the lower third of the esophagus.

D. Gastric tumors. Most gastric tumors are malignant.

1. Adenocarcinoma. Lesions may be flat and plaque-like (superficial), ulcerating and crater-like, or polypoid. Diffuse infiltration of the gastric wall is referred to as **linitis plastica** ("leather bottle stomach").

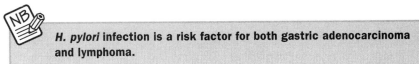

> **Superficial gastric adenocarcinomas are the only curable gastric cancers.**

2. Lymphomas arising from sites other than lymph nodes usually originate from the B cells of mucosa-associated lymphoid tissue (MALT) in the gastrointestinal tract ("MALTomas"). Within the gastrointestinal system, the stomach is the most common site of gastrointestinal lymphoma.

> ***H. pylori* infection is a risk factor for both gastric adenocarcinoma and lymphoma.**

E. Intestinal tumors

1. Small intestine. Tumors of the small intestine are the least common of all alimentary system tumors. Histologically, they are identical to colonic tumors.

2. Large intestine

a. Benign polyps (Figure 10-2) are very common. They may be solitary or multiple.

b. Colorectal adenocarcinoma is the most common alimentary system malignancy.

(1) Pathologic findings

(a) In the cecum, lesions are usually flat or ulcerated.

(b) In the rectosigmoid colon, lesions are circumferential (**"napkin ring lesions"**), leading to intestinal obstruction.

(2) Clinical findings. Hematochezia is the most common symptom. Intestinal obstruction can result in **"pencil-like" stools.** All colorectal adenocarcinomas are associated with **elevated serum carcinoembryonic antigen (CEA) levels.**

(3) Prognosis depends on the extent to which the tumor has penetrated the bowel wall and whether regional lymph node involvement or distant metastases have occurred (Dukes' classification).

c. Carcinoids are low-grade neuroendocrine tumors that secrete serotonin and neuroendocrine polypeptides. Similar tumors occur in the small intestine and appendix.

d. Lymphoma. A small percentage of gastrointestinal lymphomas arise from MALT in the large intestine.

F. Anal tumors. Squamous cell carcinoma (either *in situ* or invasive) may be seen.

> **Squamous cell carcinomas occur both at the beginning (i.e., the oral cavity and esophagus) and at the end (i.e., the anus) of the gastrointestinal tract.**

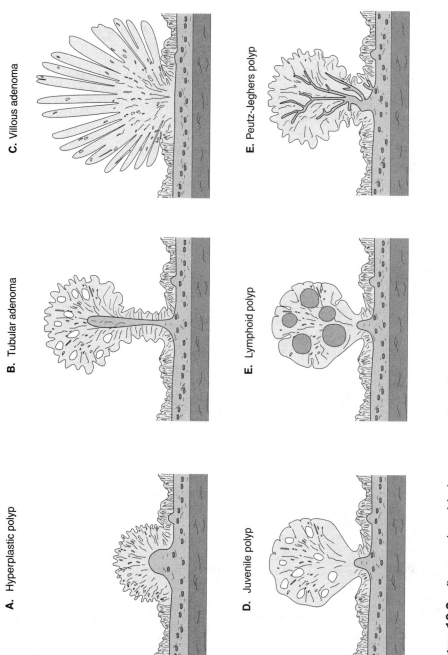

Figure 10-2. Benign polyps of the large intestine. Hyperplastic polyps (A) are common, but clinically unimportant. Tubular adenomas (B), pedunculated tumors that often occur in groups, are associated with a 2%–3% chance of malignant transformation. Villous adenomas (C), broad-based tumors composed of finger-like projections, are associated with a 40%–50% chance of malignant transformation. Juvenile polyps (D), lymphoid polyps (E), and Peutz-Jeghers polyps (F) are not associated with malignant transformation.

11

Pathology of the Liver, Biliary System, and Pancreas

I. JAUNDICE results from abnormal processing of bilirubin, one of the end-products of heme degradation. Figure 11-1 illustrates normal bilirubin metabolism.

    A. Hemolytic jaundice results from excessive production of unconjugated bilirubin, such as occurs in hemolytic anemia.

    B. Hepatocellular jaundice. Two mechanisms may be responsible for hepatocellular jaundice:

        1. Impaired hepatic uptake of unconjugated bilirubin

        2. Release of conjugated bilirubin from damaged hepatocytes (e.g., as occurs in hepatitis)

    C. Obstructive jaundice results from blocked excretion of conjugated bilirubin into the bile (e.g., as a result of extrahepatic obstruction of the common bile duct).

II. CIRRHOSIS, a synonym for **end-stage liver disease,** is characterized by a loss of normal liver architecture owing to extensive fibrosis and nodular regeneration of the liver parenchyma.

    A. Causes

        1. Alcohol abuse

        2. Chronic viral hepatitis (i.e., hepatitis B, C, or D)

        3. Autoimmune diseases (e.g., primary biliary cirrhosis, autoimmune hepatitis, sclerosing cholangitis)

        4. Hereditary disorders (e.g., α_1-antitrypsin deficiency, hemochromatosis, Wilson disease)

        5. Drug toxicity

        6. Long-standing biliary obstruction (secondary biliary cirrhosis)

> **NB** In approximately 20%–30% of patients, the cause of cirrhosis cannot be established (cryptogenic cirrhosis).

    B. Pathologic findings. In all cases, the liver is **firm,** owing to fibrosis, and **nodular.** Gross

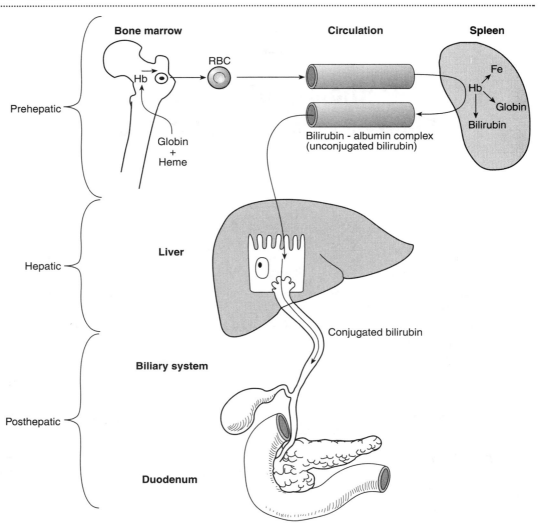

Bone marrow   **Circulation**   **Spleen**

RBC

Prehepatic

Globin
+
Heme

Fe

Hb

Globin

Bilirubin

Bilirubin - albumin complex
(unconjugated bilirubin)

Liver

Hepatic

Conjugated bilirubin

Biliary system

Posthepatic

Duodenum

Figure 11-1. Normal bilirubin metabolism and excretion. In the liver, bilirubin undergoes conjugation (i.e., the addition of glucuronic acid), which leads to the formation of water-soluble bilirubin glucuronides. The conjugated bilirubin is excreted into the bile. *Fe* = iron; *Hb* = hemoglobin; *RBC* = red blood cell.

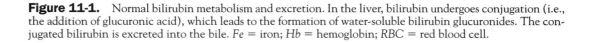

examination may allow classification of the cirrhosis as micronodular, macronodular, or irregular, but these distinctions are not clinically significant.

1. Alcoholic cirrhosis. The liver appears to be fatty (yellow) and uniformly micronodular. The liver may be enlarged, of normal size, or small.

2. Posthepatitic cirrhosis. The liver is usually shrunken, macronodular, and traversed by irregular fibrous scars. There are histologic signs of chronic inflammation.

3. Pigmentary cirrhosis is the characteristic lesion of hemochromatosis. The liver parenchyma contains nodules of variable size and is reddish-brown owing to iron pigment accumulation.

4. **Biliary cirrhosis** may be primary (caused by autoimmune destruction of the portal bile ducts) or secondary (caused by chronic biliary obstruction). In both cases, the cirrhotic liver is greenish-yellow.

5. **Cryptogenic cirrhosis.** The morphology varies. This diagnosis is made after the disorders listed in II B 1–4 and rare causes of cirrhosis (e.g., Wilson disease, α_1-antitrypsin deficiency) have been ruled out.

C. **Clinical findings.** The signs and symptoms of cirrhosis are summarized in Figure 11-2. Three major mechanisms are responsible for the clinical manifestations of cirrhosis:

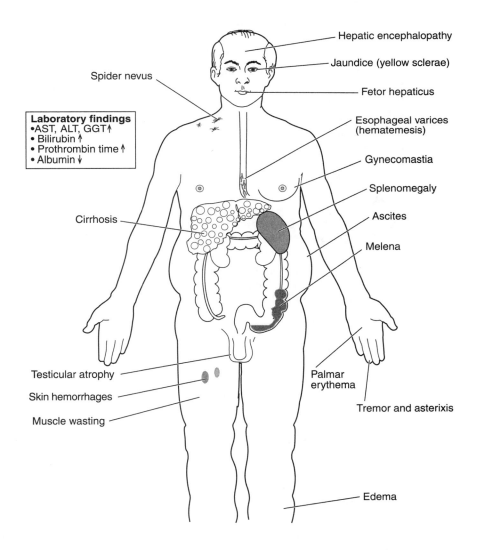

Figure 11-2.   Clinical manifestations of cirrhosis. AST = aspartate aminotransferase, ALT = alanine aminotransferase, GGT = γ-glutamyl transferase.

1. **Disturbance or loss of liver function**
   a. Impaired bilirubin conjugation leads to **hepatocellular jaundice.**
   b. Hypoalbuminemia (as a result of decreased hepatic protein synthesis) contributes to the formation of **ascites** and **edema.**
   c. Reduced production of fibrinogen, prothrombin, and other clotting factors leads to a bleeding tendency, manifested as **cutaneous** and **mucosal hemorrhages** (the latter occur on internal organs).

    All clotting factors except factor III (tissue factor), factor IV (calcium), and von Willebrand factor (vWF) are produced by the liver!

   d. Hyperestrinism (as a result of inadequate hepatic degradation of hormones) leads to **spider nevi** and **palmar erythema.** In men, the estrogen excess leads to **gynecomastia** and **testicular atrophy.**

2. **Destruction of hepatocytes.** Damaged hepatocytes release **alanine aminotransferase (ALT), aspartate aminotransferase (AST),** and **γ-glutamyl transferase (GGT),** leading to increased serum levels of these enzymes.

3. **Portal hypertension,** which has four major consequences:
   a. **Splenomegaly**
   b. **Ascites**
   c. **Portal–systemic venous shunts,** clinically manifested as **esophageal varices, caput medusae,** and **hemorrhoids**

    Bleeding from esophageal varices is a common cause of death in patients with portal hypertension.

   d. **Hepatic encephalopathy,** a metabolic disorder of the central nervous system (CNS) and neuromuscular system caused by the shunting of portal blood (containing ammonia and other toxins) to the systemic circulation

III. HEPATITIS (i.e., inflammation of the liver) may be acute or chronic. Chronic hepatitis may progress to cirrhosis.

   A. Causes

   1. **Viruses.** Hepatotropic viruses account for most hepatic infections.

    Bacterial infections of the liver cause abscesses, rather than diffuse hepatitis. Abscesses result also from amebiasis.

   2. **Drugs and toxins.** Hepatitis may be a direct effect of the drug, or a result of hypersensitivity to it.

   3. **Autoimmune diseases.** The most important in relation to hepatitis are **primary biliary cirrhosis,** which is characterized by destruction of the portal bile ducts, and **autoimmune hepatitis.**

   B. Pathologic findings

  1. Acute hepatitis. Findings include:
   a. **Intralobular** and **portal tract infiltrates** of lymphocytes and macrophages
   b. **Ballooning degeneration** (i.e., diffuse swelling of hepatocytes)
   c. **Apoptotic hepatocytes (Councilman bodies),** which are shrunken and intensely eosinophilic with fragmented nuclei
   d. **Kupffer cell hyperplasia** and **hypertrophy**
   e. **Regenerative changes**

> **Massive hepatic necrosis, a rare complication of hepatitis B (and less often, other forms of viral hepatitis) is characterized by widespread liver cell necrosis.**

  2. Chronic hepatitis. Findings include:
   a. **Intralobular** and **portal tract inflammation**
   b. **Piecemeal (periportal) necrosis,** as a result of inflammatory "spillover" from the portal tracts to the adjacent parenchyma
   c. **Bridging necrosis** and the formation of **connective tissue septa** between adjacent portal tracts (an ominous sign indicative of progression to cirrhosis)

C. Clinical diagnosis

  1. **Symptoms** are usually nonspecific (e.g., **nausea, jaundice, liver tenderness**).

  2. **Laboratory studies** are essential and reveal elevated blood levels of bilirubin, ALT, and AST.
   a. **Acute viral hepatitis** is diagnosed using serologic studies.
   b. **Chronic hepatitis.** Biochemical findings are variable and depend on the extent and activity of the disease.
    (1) **Antimitochondrial antibodies (AMA)** are a sign of primary biliary cirrhosis.
    (2) **Antinuclear antibodies (ANA)** and **anti-smooth muscle antibodies (ASMA)** are signs of autoimmune hepatitis.
   c. **Liver biopsy.** Although not particularly useful for determining the cause of hepatitis, liver biopsy is performed in chronic hepatitis to determine the extent of injury and to evaluate the progression of disease.

IV. TOXIC OR METABOLIC LIVER INJURY

A. Causes

  1. **Inborn errors of metabolism** that cause liver damage include α_1-**antitrypsin deficiency, hemochromatosis** (characterized by excessive iron deposition in parenchymal organs) and **Wilson disease** (characterized by excessive copper deposition in the liver, brain, and eye).

  2. **Alcohol abuse** causes **hepatic steatosis (fatty liver),** which is clinically insignificant. However, 15%–20% of patients with alcoholism develop either **alcoholic hepatitis** or **cirrhosis.**

  3. **Drugs.** The effect of drugs may be predictable (i.e., dose related) or unpredictable (i.e., idiosyncratic hypersensitivity). For example, an overdose of acetaminophen is invariably associated with liver cell necrosis, but only some patients taking diuretics or psychoactive drugs develop liver injury.

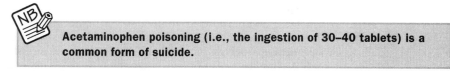

Acetaminophen poisoning (i.e., the ingestion of 30–40 tablets) is a common form of suicide.

    4. Toxins. Many poisons damage the liver in a predictable, dose-related manner (e.g., mushroom poisoning, phosphorus poisoning).

  B. Pathologic findings. Acute liver injury may present as focal or widespread liver cell necrosis. When the injury is chronic, fibrosis is seen, and possibly progression to cirrhosis.

    1. Alcoholic liver disease. The liver shows **fatty change** and **Mallory bodies** (i.e., cytoplasmic aggregates of intermediate filaments bound by ubiquitin).

    2. Acetaminophen toxicity causes **centrilobular necrosis.**

    3. Isoniazid toxicity produces **histopathologic features similar to those of hepatitis.**

    4. Chlorpromazine toxicity is characterized by **cholestasis** (i.e., the formation of "bile plugs" between hepatocytes).

  C. Clinical diagnosis is usually based on:

    1. A history of exposure

    2. Laboratory signs of liver injury

    3. Liver biopsy results

    4. Clinical improvement following removal of the offending agent

V. BILIARY OBSTRUCTION results in **jaundice, conjugated hyperbilirubinemia,** and **clay-colored (acholic) stools.** Long-lasting biliary obstruction causes secondary biliary cirrhosis.

  A. Intrahepatic causes include the following:

    1. Primary biliary cirrhosis, an autoimmune disease that results in destruction of the portal bile ducts

    2. Primary sclerosing cholangitis, an inflammatory disease often associated with inflammatory bowel disease (IBD) that involves both the intrahepatic and the extrahepatic bile ducts

    3. Cholangitis (i.e., acute inflammation of the bile duct wall, usually caused by bacterial infection)

    4. Cirrhosis

  B. Extrahepatic causes are illustrated in Figure 11-3.

VI. CHOLELITHIASIS. Gallstones may be found in the gallbladder or biliary ducts.

  A. Types of gallstones

    1. Cholesterol stones are **yellow** and are typically found in overweight, older women (think of the **"four Fs": female, fat, fertile, and over forty).**

    2. Pigment stones are **brown** or **black** stones composed of bilirubin salts.
      a. Black pigment stones are seen most often in patients with **hemolytic diseases** (e.g., sickle cell anemia).

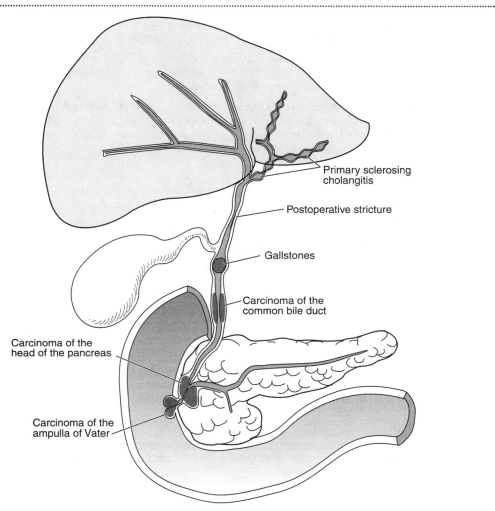

Figure 11-3. Extrahepatic causes of biliary obstruction.

        b. **Brown pigment stones** are rare in the United States but common in Asia. **Cholangitis** predisposes to the development of brown pigment stones.

    B. **Complications of cholelithiasis** include:

        1. **Cholecystitis** (i.e., inflammation of the gallbladder). In chronic cholecystitis, the gallbladder is thick and calcified **("porcelain gallbladder").**

        2. **Obstruction of the cystic duct** causes biliary colic (i.e., spasmodic pain).

        3. **Obstruction of the common bile duct** leads to jaundice, pancreatitis, or both.

VII. **PANCREATITIS** may be acute or chronic.

    A. **Causes.** Pancreatitis is usually a sterile (i.e., noninfectious) inflammation.

1. **Mild interstitial pancreatitis** accompanies many systemic diseases and is of no clinical significance.

2. **Acute hemorrhagic pancreatitis**, a potentially lethal disease, is related to **alcohol abuse** or **gallstones** in 80% of cases. Other, less common, causes include **trauma, drugs, infection,** and **metabolic disorders.**

3. **Chronic pancreatitis** is a disease associated with **alcoholism** (90% of patients). In approximately 50% of these patients, chronic pancreatitis is preceded by at least one bout of acute pancreatitis. Chronic pancreatitis may also be a consequence of **cystic fibrosis.**

B. Pathologic findings

1. **Interstitial pancreatitis** is characterized by edema and interstitial inflammation. Computed tomography (CT) reveals an enlarged pancreas.

2. **Acute hemorrhagic pancreatitis** is characterized by extensive hemorrhage into a swollen, necrotic pancreas.
   a. The release of **pancreatic enzymes** (i.e., **amylase, lipase** and the protease **trypsin**) causes tissue destruction (i.e., **fat necrosis**) and **ascites.**
   b. **Pancreatic pseudocyst**, a late complication of acute hemorrhagic pancreatitis, occurs when fibrotic tissue surrounds areas of necrotic pancreatic parenchyma. The walled-off cavity contains enzymes and liquefied tissue.

3. **Chronic pancreatitis** is characterized by a **shrunken, firm, fibrotic pancreas** with **calcifications.**

C. Clinical findings

1. **Acute hemorrhagic pancreatitis.** Signs and symptoms include **severe abdominal pain, vomiting, upper quadrant tenderness,** and **ascites.** Vascular collapse may cause **shock.**

> **Serum amylase and lipase levels become elevated 24–72 hours after the onset of the attack.**

2. **Chronic pancreatitis.** Clinical manifestations include **epigastric pain** (which may be unrelenting), **malabsorption** (owing to a lack of pancreatic enzymes), **diabetes** (as a result of islet cell destruction), and **calcifications** (visible radiographically).

VIII. NEOPLASMS OF THE LIVER, BILIARY SYSTEM, AND PANCREAS

A. Carcinoma of the liver

> **The most common malignant tumor of the liver is metastasis from other sites. Metastatic tumors form multiple nodules.**

1. **Types of primary liver cancer**
   a. **Hepatocellular carcinoma** is rare in the United States; however, worldwide, it is one of the most common malignant tumors. Hepatocellular carcinoma is responsible for millions of deaths in Africa and Asia, where the incidence of chronic viral hepatitis (i.e., hepatitis B, C, or D) is higher (demonstrating a link between the two disorders).

    b. Cholangiocarcinoma (adenocarcinoma of bile duct origin) is rare in the United States. The incidence is higher in China, where the liver fluke *Opisthorchis sinensis* is endemic.

  2. Pathologic findings. The neoplastic cells in hepatocellular carcinoma resemble liver cells. Most tumors originate in cirrhotic livers.

  3. Clinical findings include **pain** (resulting from the distention of nerves in the Glisson capsule), **hepatic enlargement** (possibly palpable), and **paraneoplastic syndromes** (e.g., hypoglycemia, erythrocytosis). **α-Fetoprotein (AFP)** is a tumor marker for hepatocellular carcinoma that is detectable in the blood.

> **Benign liver cell adenomas occur in young women and are associated with oral contraceptive use. These tumors contain numerous vessels and may bleed, especially during pregnancy.**

B. **Carcinoma of the gallbladder** is rare in the United States. Typically, patients are elderly women with gallstones.

  1. Pathologic findings. In 90% of cases, the neoplasm is an adenocarcinoma; the remaining cases are squamous cell carcinomas originating from squamous metaplasia as a result of chronic irritation by gallstones.

  2. Clinical findings. The **pain** of gallbladder carcinoma is indistinguishable from that of cholecystitis or cholelithiasis.

C. **Carcinoma of the pancreas** is the fourth most common cause of cancer-related death in men in the United States (fifth in women). The incidence of this cancer has tripled within the past 50 years.

  1. Pathologic findings. Adenocarcinomas originating from the pancreatic ducts account for 90% of cases.

  2. Clinical findings in pancreatic cancer include:
    a. **Pain that radiates to the back**
    b. A **mass** (best visualized by CT)
    c. **Jaundice** (owing to obstruction or compression of the bile duct)
    d. **Paraneoplastic syndromes** (e.g., **Trousseau syndrome,** characterized by migrating thrombophlebitis)
    e. **Carcinoembryonic antigen (CEA),** a tumor marker for all adenocarcinomas, including those of hepatobiliary and pancreatic origin

D. **Islet cell tumors** are rare pancreatic tumors of low malignant potential. These tumors are classified according to their cellular composition as **insulinomas** (β cells), **glucagonomas** (α cells), **gastrinomas,** or **vasointestinal polypeptide–secreting tumors (VIPomas).**

  1. Pathologic findings. Histologically these tumors have "neuroendocrine features" and resemble carcinoids. They contain granules visible by electron microscopy and stain immunohistochemically with antibodies to chromogranin.

  2. Clinical findings include **hypoglycemia** (insulinomas), **mild diabetes** and **migratory necrotizing dermatitis** (glucagonomas), **Zollinger-Ellison syndrome** (gastrinomas), and **watery diarrhea** (VIPomas). Polypeptide hormones (e.g. insulin, glucagon) produced by islet cell tumors can be readily measured in the blood.

12

Pathology of the Kidneys and Urinary Tract

I. **DEVELOPMENTAL DISORDERS** may be major and evident at birth or during infancy, or minor and asymptomatic. Some disorders [e.g., autosomal dominant polycystic kidney disease (ADPKD)] produce symptoms only later in life.

A. **Renal agenesis**

1. Agenesis of **one kidney** occurs in 1 of 800 births and is usually asymptomatic.

2. Agenesis of **both kidneys (Potter syndrome)** occurs in 1 of 5000 births and is lethal.

B. **Horseshoe kidney,** which occurs when the kidneys fail to separate at the lower pole during development, may cause compression of the vena cava or aorta.

C. **Ectopic kidney.** Abnormal upward migration of the fetal kidneys results in positional anomalies. Ectopic kidneys are most often located in the pelvis and are prone to infection or obstruction.

D. **Renal cystic disease** results from abnormal differentiation of metanephric blastema.

1. **Multicystic renal dysplasia.** Cysts are embedded in a connective tissue stroma formed of heterotopic tissue (e.g., cartilage). Multicystic renal dysplasia usually presents as a one-sided renal mass.

> **A palpable abdominal mass in an infant usually represents one of three conditions: multicystic renal dysplasia, Wilms tumor, or neuroblastoma of the adrenal gland.**

2. **Autosomal dominant polycystic kidney disease (ADPKD),** caused by an abnormality in two genes, occurs in 1 out of 1000 births. Typically, there is bilateral enlargement of the kidneys, which contain numerous fluid-filled cysts and weigh more than 1000 grams each. Renal failure occurs during **adulthood.**

3. **Autosomal recessive polycystic kidney disease (ARPKD)** is less common than ADPKD. In ARPKD, the kidneys contain small cysts and are only slightly enlarged. Renal failure occurs during **infancy.**

II. **GLOMERULONEPHRITIS.** In all forms of glomerulonephritis, the **deposition of immune complexes within the glomeruli** leads to **inflammation.** The inflammatory response may cause proliferation of endothelial, mesangial, and epithelial cells and, in severe disease, glomerular necrosis. Clinically, glomerular inflammation causes **nephritic**

syndrome, which comprises edema, proteinuria, hypoalbuminemia, hematuria, and hypertension.

A. Proliferative glomerulonephritis

1. **Acute poststreptococcal glomerulonephritis** typically is a sequela of "strep throat," developing 2–4 weeks after the initial infection. Most patients are children who recover spontaneously; only 1%–2% of patients progress to chronic glomerulonephritis.

a. **Pathologic findings** (Figure 12-1) include **hypercellular glomeruli** containing inflammatory cells (e.g., neutrophils, macrophages) and an increased number of mesangial and endothelial cells. **Subepithelial immune complexes** ("isolated humps") are seen by electron microscopy.

b. **Clinical findings.** Clinically, acute poststreptococcal glomerulonephritis presents as a **short-lived nephritic syndrome,** characterized by **edema, proteinuria, oliguria, brown urine (hematuria),** and **hypertension.**

2. **IgA nephropathy (Berger disease)** is the most common form of glomerulonephritis. It may occur after infection, but its pathogenesis is unknown.

a. **Pathologic findings** include **focal mesangial cell proliferation** and **mesangial deposits of IgA** (seen by electron microscopy or immunofluorescence microscopy).

b. **Clinical findings.** The presentation may vary from mild hematuria and proteinuria to slowly progressive renal failure. Patients do not respond to therapy with immunosuppressive drugs or steroids.

3. **Lupus nephritis** is found in 75% of patients with systemic lupus erythematosus (SLE). Usually, the inflammation can be treated with corticosteroids and cyclophosphamide. However, approximately 20% of patients present with membranous nephropathy, which is resistant to treatment.

a. **Pathologic findings** include **hypercellular glomeruli** with **"wire loop" thickening** of the basement membranes. **Immune complex deposits** vary in size and may be found in any portion of the glomerulus.

b. **Clinical findings.** The presentation varies from mild hematuria and proteinuria to signs of severe renal dysfunction. Antinuclear antibodies (ANA) and other clinical manifestations of SLE are evident.

B. **Crescentic glomerulonephritis** occurs as a consequence of focal necrotizing glomerulonephritis. Following rupture of the damaged glomerular capillary loops, an inflammatory exudate containing macrophages fills the glomerular urinary space. The inflammatory exudate, along with proliferation of the epithelial cells that line the Bowman capsule, forms a "crescent" (Figure 12-2). **Rapidly progressive glomerulonephritis (RPGN)** ensues, leading to acute renal failure.

1. **Goodpasture syndrome** is caused by an anti-glomerular basement membrane (anti-GBM) antibody that reacts with alveolar and glomerular basement membranes, leading to pulmonary hemorrhage and glomerulonephritis. Binding of the autoantibodies directly to the glomerular basement membrane results in a linear pattern on immunofluorescence microscopy staining (as opposed to the granular pattern seen in other forms of glomerulonephritis).

2. **Wegener granulomatosis** is characterized by granulomatous vasculitis and thrombosis-related infarcts in the upper respiratory tract and lungs. The glomeruli show no immune deposits, but a cytoplasmic antineutrophilic cytoplasmic antibody (c-ANCA) test is positive.

III. **GLOMERULOPATHY** is a noncommittal term applied to diseases that produce signs of glomerular disease but show no inflammation. These diseases cause **nephrotic syndrome,** which comprises edema, proteinuria, hypoalbuminemia, and hyperlipidemia.

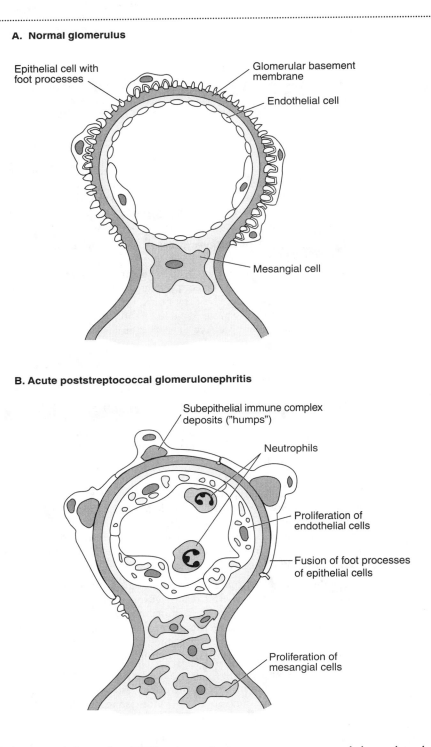

A. Normal glomerulus

Epithelial cell with foot processes

Glomerular basement membrane

Endothelial cell

Mesangial cell

B. Acute poststreptococcal glomerulonephritis

Subepithelial immune complex deposits ("humps")

Neutrophils

Proliferation of endothelial cells

Fusion of foot processes of epithelial cells

Proliferation of mesangial cells

Figure 12-1. (A) A normal glomerulus. (B) The glomerulus in acute poststreptococcal glomerulonephritis.

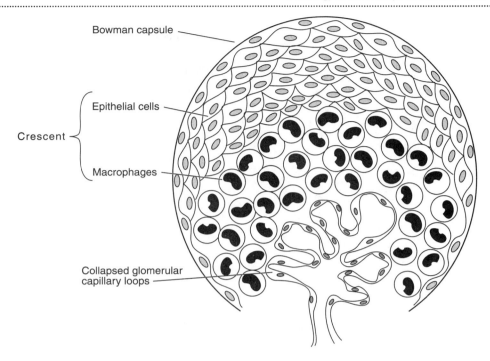

Figure 12-2.   Crescentic glomerulonephritis.

A. Membranous nephropathy, the most common primary renal cause of nephrotic syndrome in adults, is characterized by **subepithelial "lumpy-bumpy" (granular) immune complex deposits** (Figure 12-3). The disorder does not respond to treatment and will progress to end-stage renal failure over a period of 12–15 years.

   1. Primary membranous nephropathy is idiopathic.

   2. Secondary membranous nephropathy is seen in some patients with SLE, cancer, or infections (e.g., viral hepatitis). In these patients, the nephropathy may be related to circulating antigen–antibody complexes (e.g., those formed from tumor antigens or hepatitis virus B or C antigens).

B. Minimal change disease (lipoid nephrosis), the most common cause of nephrotic syndrome in children, is a disease of unknown etiology that affects mostly children. By light and immunofluorescence microscopy, the glomeruli appear normal, but electron microscopy shows fusion of the foot processes. Patients respond well to corticosteroid therapy.

C. Focal segmental glomerulosclerosis is a disease of unknown etiology that involves only some of the glomeruli (hence the designation "focal") and is characterized by hyalinization (sclerosis) of parts of those glomeruli (hence the designation "segmental"). The disorder may be idiopathic or secondary to a systemic disease (e.g., AIDS) and is unresponsive to therapy.

D. Glomerulopathies of nonimmune origin are encountered in two systemic diseases, diabetes mellitus and amyloidosis.

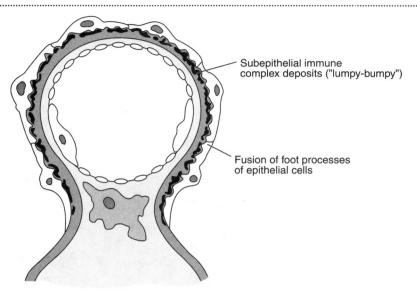

Subepithelial immune
complex deposits ("lumpy-bumpy")

Fusion of foot processes
of epithelial cells

Figure 12-3.   Membranous nephropathy.

1. Diabetic glomerulopathy occurs in two forms, diffuse or nodular (Kimmelstiel-Wilson disease). Diabetic glomerulopathy is the most common cause of nephrotic syndrome.

2. Amyloidosis may be a feature of multiple myeloma (primary amyloidosis) or a complication of chronic suppurative disease (secondary amyloidosis).

 Uremia (i.e., end-stage kidney disease) may ensue over time from any glomerular disease.

IV. TUBULOINTERSTITIAL NEPHRITIS

A. Acute (allergic) tubulointerstitial nephritis is most often caused by a type IV hypersensitivity (cell-mediated) reaction to therapeutic drugs. Pathologically, it is characterized by tubular injury and renal interstitial infiltrates containing T lymphocytes, macrophages, and eosinophils. Patients present with acute renal failure.

B. Chronic (immune-mediated) tubulointerstitial nephritis is a typical feature of chronic renal transplant rejection.

V. URINARY TRACT INFECTIONS (UTIs). The route of infection may be either **hematogenous** (e.g., in patients with sepsis, septic emboli, or endocarditis) or **ascending.** Factors that predispose to ascending UTIs are shown in Figure 12-4.

 UTIs are diagnosed clinically and confirmed by urinalysis, which shows bacterial colonies in excess of 100,000/ml and leukocyturia.

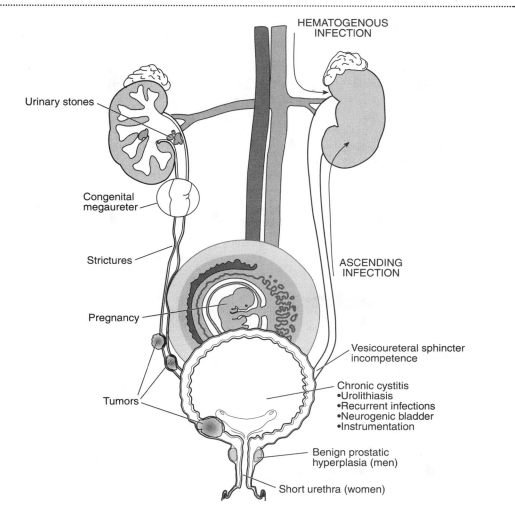

Figure 12-4.   Factors that predispose to ascending urinary tract infections (UTIs).

A. Urethritis, the most common UTI, may be caused by sexually transmitted pathogens (e.g., *Neisseria gonorrhoeae, Chlamydia trachomatis*) or Gram-negative uropathogens (e.g., *Escherichia coli, Pseudomonas aeruginosa*). Patients complain of urinary urgency, burning during urination, and a urethral discharge.

B. Cystitis is usually a complication of urethritis, but it may occur as a primary disease following instrumentation (e.g. catheterization, cystoscopy), urinary obstruction (e.g., benign prostatic hyperplasia), or bladder irritation (e.g., as a result of urolithiasis). Patients present with urgency, dysuria, and hematuria; bacteria and leukocytes can be detected in the urine.

C. Ureteritis may occur as a result of vesicoureteral reflux and may progress to pyelonephritis. The congenital defect predisposing to vesicoureteral reflux is found in 2%–3% of patients and is an important cause of UTI in young girls and women.

D. Pyelonephritis is a term used for bacterial infections of the kidneys, renal calices, and pelves.

> **To remember the Gram-negative uropathogens most often responsible for pyelonephritis, remember the mnemonic KEEPS:**
> *Klebsiella*
> *Escherichia coli*
> *Enterobacter*
> *Proteus*
> *Serratia*

1. **Acute pyelonephritis** is a purulent infection that may involve one or both kidneys. Patients present with flank pain, fever, and dysuria.

2. **Chronic pyelonephritis** is caused by protracted or recurrent infections. Pathologically, chronic pyelonephritis is characterized by irregular scarring of the kidney, deformities of the collecting system, hydronephrosis, and loss of the renal parenchyma. Complications include:
   a. **End-stage kidney disease,** in patients with bilateral involvement
   b. **Papillary necrosis,** which may cause **urinary colics** owing to obstruction of the ureters by sloughed papillae

VI. CIRCULATORY DISORDERS

A. **Ischemic acute tubular necrosis (ATN)** is a common consequence of renal hypoperfusion in patients with **hypovolemic** or **endotoxemic shock** or **circulatory collapse** owing to pump failure (e.g., myocardial infarct). Tubular necrosis leads to oliguria; however, the oliguria is reversible, because the tubules regenerate. Patients placed on dialysis survive and enter a polyuric phase before fully recovering. The urine contains dark brown granular casts.

B. **Bilateral renal cortical necrosis** is a complication of **eclampsia and abruptio placentae, postpartum bleeding,** or **endotoxic shock.**

C. **Chronic renal ischemia** results from **atherosclerosis** and is characterized by hyalinization of glomeruli, tubular atrophy and loss, and interstitial fibrosis. The kidneys are small, shrunken, and may be afunctional. Chronic renal ischemia is an important cause of end-stage kidney disease among the elderly.

VII. TOXIC OR METABOLIC RENAL INJURY

A. **Nephrotoxic ATN** results from poisoning with **heavy metals** (e.g., mercury), **organophosphorous compounds,** and some **therapeutic drugs** (e.g., **gentamycin**).

B. **Diabetic nephropathy.** Diabetes mellitus predisposes the patient to:

   1. **Glomerulosclerosis,** leading to nephrotic syndrome

   2. **Arteriosclerosis,** leading to renal ischemia and hypertension

   3. **Pyelonephritis** (a result of hyperglycemia of the interstitial tissues, which facilitates bacterial infection)

   4. **Papillary necrosis**

C. **Hyperuricemia** leads to deposits of uric acid in the renal parenchyma and tubules, and urolithiasis.

D. Urolithiasis is a common disease; 5%–10% of the population is affected over the course of a lifetime. Men are affected more often than women.

    1. Types of urinary stones

        a. Calcium oxalate and **calcium phosphate stones** account for 75% of uroliths. Hypercalciuria and hyperuricosuria are the main risk factors for the development of these stones.

        b. Struvite stones ("staghorn calculi") are ammonium magnesium phosphate stones that form in alkaline urine, such as occurs in patients with persistent UTIs. Struvite stones are found in 15% of patients with urolithiasis.

        c. Uric acid stones (found in 9% of patients) are typically seen in association with gout, but in 50% cases they occur without hyperuricemia.

        d. Cystine stones (found in 1% of patients) occur in patients with cystinosis, an inborn error of metabolism.

    2. Complications of urolithiasis include

        a. Urinary colics (owing to impaction in the ureter)

        b. Hydroureter and **hydronephrosis** (owing to obstruction of urinary outflow)

        c. Infection (related to mucosal injury and obstruction)

VIII. NEOPLASMS OF THE KIDNEYS AND URINARY TRACT (Figure 12-5)

A. Tumors of the kidneys

    1. Wilms tumor (nephroblastoma) is a malignant tumor originating from the renal blastema. Its peak incidence is in children between the ages of 1 and 3 years. Following surgery combined with chemotherapy, the 5-year survival rate is greater than 90%.

    2. Renal cell carcinoma, derived from renal tubular cells, is the most common renal tumor in adults. This neoplasm is typically seen in men between the ages of 50 and 70 years. The tumor, which is resistant to chemotherapy, is associated with a 5-year survival rate of 45%.

        a. Clinical findings. Symptoms vary (hence the nickname **"internist's tumor"**); the classic triad of hematuria, flank pain, and a mass is found in only 10% of patients.

        b. Complications include hematogenous **metastasis,** following invasion of the renal veins.

    3. Transitional cell carcinoma of the renal pelvis. Small, well-differentiated tumors are associated with a 5-year survival rate of 70%, but undifferentiated tumors are more malignant.

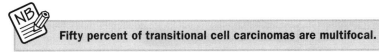

        Fifty percent of transitional cell carcinomas are multifocal.

B. Tumors of the urinary bladder are the most common type of urinary tract tumor. In 90% of cases, they are **transitional cell carcinomas;** the remaining cases are **squamous cell carcinomas** or **adenocarcinomas.** Typically, patients are men between the ages of 50 and 80 years.

    1. Predisposing factors include cigarette smoking and exposure to aniline dyes.

    2. Clinical findings include hematuria; dysuria; and a mass effect in the pelvic region, at sites of metastasis, or both.

    3. Treatment is surgical, but may include adjuvant therapy with cytotoxic drugs and intravesical bacille Calmette-Guérin (BCG) immunotherapy.

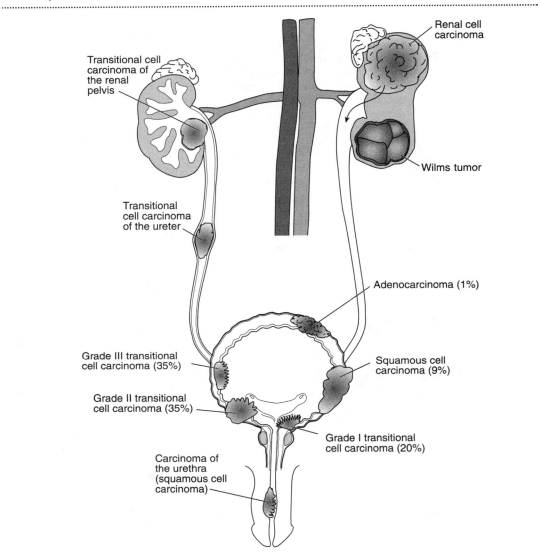

Figure 12-5. Neoplasms of the urinary tract.

4. Prognosis depends on the histologic grade: the 5-year survival rate ranges from 90% for patients with grade I disease to 30% for patients with grade III disease.

C. Tumors of the ureters and urethra. Transitional cell carcinomas in these locations are rare. Obstruction is an early symptom.

13

Pathology of the Male Reproductive System

I. DEVELOPMENTAL DISORDERS

- **A. Cryptorchidism (undescended testis),** found in 0.5% of male infants, predisposes to testicular tumors and, if bilateral, may cause infertility.

- **B. Hypospadias.** The urethral opening is located on the ventral aspect of the penile shaft.

- **C. Epispadias.** The urethral opening is located on the dorsal aspect of the penile shaft.

  - **1.** Epispadias is less common than hypospadias.

  - **2.** Epispadias may be associated with urinary bladder anomalies (e.g., exstrophy).

- **D. Phimosis.** Narrowing of the preputium prevents its retraction over the glans penis.

II. INFECTIONS OF THE MALE REPRODUCTIVE TRACT. The route of infection is most often ascending, but may be hematogenous. In young men, most infections are sexually transmitted, whereas in elderly men, infections are usually related to urinary obstruction by the prostate.

- **A. Orchitis** (i.e., infection of the testis) may be viral (e.g., mumps) or bacterial.

- **B. Epididymitis** is almost always related to ascending bacterial infection.

> **Epididymoorchitis is the most common intrascrotal infection because the infection often spreads from one structure to the other.**

- **C. Prostatitis.** Bacterial infection of the prostate is common among elderly patients. However, symptoms are usually overshadowed by signs of urinary obstruction.

- **D. Urethritis** is usually caused by *Neisseria gonorrhoeae*, *Chlamydia trachomatis*, or mixed bacterial flora.

> **"Nonbacterial urethritis" is a term used when no bacteria are found on a standard urine culture. In this case, the urethritis may be chlamydial or viral in origin or part of Reiter syndrome (a syndrome of unknown etiology characterized by the triad of urethritis, arthritis, and uveitis).**

- **E. Balanoposthitis** (i.e., inflammation of the glans penis) may be caused by bacteria (e.g.,

Treponema pallidum), viruses [e.g., herpes simplex virus (HSV)], or fungi (e.g., *Candida albicans*; common in patients with diabetes).

III. BENIGN PROSTATIC HYPERPLASIA (BPH), characterized by non-neoplastic nodular hyperplasia of the prostatic glands and stroma, is the most common cause of prostatic enlargement in elderly men. The cause of BPH is not known, but the condition may be related to an androgen/estrogen imbalance that occurs in old age.

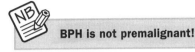

BPH is not premalignant!

A. **Pathologic findings.** Nodule formation occurs predominantly in the middle lobe and periurethral portion of the prostate.

B. **Clinical findings.** Patients have symptoms related to urethral compression (e.g., urgency) and urinary bladder obstruction [e.g., recurrent urinary tract infections (UTIs)]. On rectal digital examination, the enlarged prostate is soft.

C. **Complications** include hypertrophy and hyperplasia of the urinary bladder ("trabeculation"), UTI, and hydronephrosis (in patients with prolonged obstruction).

D. **Treatment.** The nodular hyperplasia can be "shelled out" from the peripherally compressed prostatic tissue (the so-called "surgical capsule").

IV. NEOPLASMS OF THE MALE REPRODUCTIVE TRACT

A. Tumors of the testis

1. **Germ cell tumors** account for 95% of all testicular tumors. The peak incidence of these tumors is between the ages of 25 and 40 years. Although most germ cell tumors are malignant, they are curable in 90% of cases.

a. **Seminomas** are the most common testicular tumor (45% of cases).
   (1) **Pathologic findings.** Seminomas are composed of a single cell type (clear cells, similar to spermatogonia) arranged into lobules surrounded by septa that contain lymphocytes.
   (2) **Clinical findings** include painless enlargement of the testis. Seminomas do not secrete tumor markers.
   (3) **Treatment.** Surgery and radiation therapy will cure 90% of patients because seminomas are extremely radiosensitive.

b. **Nonseminomatous germ cell tumors (NSGCTs)** are more malignant than seminomas. Although the primary tumors are small, metastases occur early to the abdominal lymph nodes and are often widespread (e.g., to the lungs or liver).
   (1) **Pathologic findings.** NSGCTs typically have multiple histologic patterns (Figure 13-1).
   (2) **Clinical findings.** α-Fetoprotein (AFP) and **human chorionic gonadotropin (hCG)** are detectable in the blood in 80% of cases.

Pure yolk sac carcinoma is an AFP-secreting tumor that occurs in children younger than 4 years.

   (3) **Treatment** involves surgery, abdominal lymph node dissection, and chemotherapy based on cisplatin combination regimens.

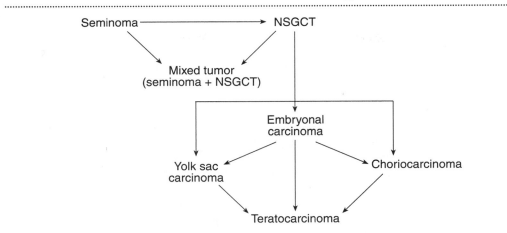

Figure 13-1. Germ cell tumors of the testis. Nonseminomatous germ cell tumors (NSGCTs) include embryonal carcinomas, yolk sac carcinomas, choriocarcinomas, and teratocarcinomas. The neoplastic cells of embryonal carcinomas may differentiate along somatic cell lines (into teratocarcinomas), or along extraembryonic cell lines (into yolk sac carcinomas or choriocarcinomas). The histologic types of NSGCTs are usually intermixed; in 15% of patients, seminomas are present as well (mixed tumors). Pure choriocarcinoma is extremely rare (1:1000 cases) but highly malignant.

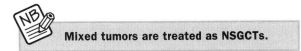

Mixed tumors are treated as NSGCTs.

    c. **Benign teratomas** are very rare in men (as opposed to those in women, where they represent the most common germ cell tumor).

  2. **Sex cord cell tumors.** Leydig cell tumors and Sertoli cell tumors are rare, accounting for only 5% of testicular tumors. These tumors can occur in any age group.

    a. **Leydig cell tumors** are hormonally active in 70% of cases. They secrete **androgens,** leading to precocious puberty in boys, or **estrogens,** leading to gynecomastia in adults.

    b. **Sertoli cell tumors** are usually hormonally inactive, but may secrete **inhibin.**

B. **Carcinoma of the prostate** is the most common malignant tumor in men. This tumor has a high prevalence in older men; generally, 30% of 50-year-old men and 60% of 80-year-old men have asymptomatic **histologic** prostatic cancer.

  1. **Pathologic findings.** Tumors are **adenocarcinomas** that originate preferentially in the glandular epithelium of the peripheral zones of the prostate and typically involve the **posterior lobe.**

  2. **Clinical findings.** The tumor causes induration of the prostate that can be palpated through the rectum. **Prostate-specific antigen (PSA)** is a useful tumor marker.

PSA levels may be elevated in patients with BPH and may be normal in those with undifferentiated prostatic carcinoma!

3. Grading. Transrectal needle biopsy is essential for diagnosis and grading according to the Gleason grading system.

    a. High-grade, poorly differentiated adenocarcinomas grow and metastasize faster than low-grade, well-differentiated tumors. Metastases may be local (i.e., in the pelvic organs and sacral vertebrae), as well as distant.

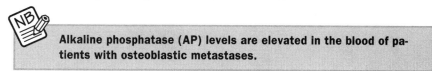 **Alkaline phosphatase (AP) levels are elevated in the blood of patients with osteoblastic metastases.**

    b. The tumor grade is the most important predictor of survival after prostatectomy. A-stage tumors are associated with a 5-year survival rate of 90%, whereas D-stage tumors carry only a 20% 5-year survival rate.

4. Treatment. Chemotherapy is ineffective, and prostatectomy is helpful only when the tumor is of a low grade and limited to the prostate.

C. Carcinoma of the penis. In the United States, squamous cell carcinoma of the penis accounts for only 0.5% of all cancers in men; this tumor is more common in South America and Africa. The prognosis depends on the stage, but overall, the 5-year survival rate is 60%.

14

Pathology of the Female Reproductive System and Breast

I. INFECTIONS OF THE FEMALE REPRODUCTIVE TRACT (Figure 14-1)

A. Vulvitis. Viruses invade epithelial cells.

1. Herpes simplex virus (HSV) causes vulvar vesicles.

2. Human papilloma virus (HPV) causes genital warts (condylomata acuminatum).

B. Vaginitis is a chronic infection most often caused by *Trichomonas vaginalis, Candida albicans,* or *Gardnerella vaginalis.* The epithelium of vagina is resistant to bacterial, fungal, and protozoal invasion; the pathogens remain intraluminal.

C. Cervicitis

1. Bacterial cervicitis. Endocervicitis is the most common presentation of gonorrhea and other bacterial infections.

2. Viral cervicitis. HSV and HPV invade the squamous epithelium of the ectocervix. Most often, the lesions present as flat papillomas.
  a. HSV infection is characterized by intranuclear inclusions ("ground glass" appearance) and multinucleation.
  b. HPV infection causes koilocytic changes.

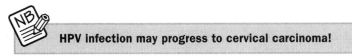

HPV infection may progress to cervical carcinoma!

D. Endometritis is uncommon during the reproductive years because of monthly endometrial shedding.

1. When present, endometritis is usually sexually transmitted and associated with pelvic inflammatory disease (PID), although it may be a complication of septic abortion or childbirth (puerperal endometritis).

2. Endometritis causes infertility. When it occurs as a complication of septic abortion, endometritis may be fatal.

E. Salpingitis, which almost always occurs as a component of PID, is the most common infection of the internal female genital organs. The fallopian tubes are tortuous ("retortlike") and contain pus. Adhesions extending to the rectum or urinary bladder are common.

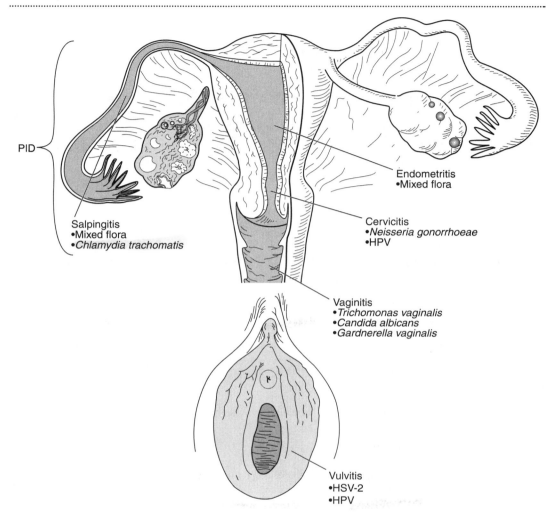

PID

Salpingitis
•Mixed flora
•*Chlamydia trachomatis*

Endometritis
•Mixed flora

Cervicitis
•*Neisseria gonorrhoeae*
•HPV

Vaginitis
•*Trichomonas vaginalis*
•*Candida albicans*
•*Gardnerella vaginalis*

Vulvitis
•HSV-2
•HPV

Figure 14-1.   Infections of the female reproductive tract. Infection may be sexually or non-sexually transmitted, acute or chronic, localized or widespread [e.g., pelvic inflammatory disease (*PID*), which encompasses endometritis, salpingitis, endocervicitis, parovarian abscesses, and pelvic peritonitis]. *HPV* = human papilloma virus; *HSV-2* = herpes simplex virus, type 2.

F. Pelvic inflammatory disease (PID), which comprises endometritis, salpingitis, parovarian abscesses, and pelvic peritonitis, is a major public health problem—in the United States, more than 2 billion dollars are spent annually for the diagnosis and treatment of PID. Infertility is a major complication.

1. Most cases of PID are sexually transmitted.

2. Clinical findings include pelvic pain and systemic signs of persistent bacterial infection.

II. HORMONALLY INDUCED DISORDERS OF THE FEMALE REPRODUCTIVE TRACT

A. **Endometrial hyperplasia** is a consequence of hyperestrinism, which may be exogenous (e.g., as a result of hormone therapy) or endogenous (e.g., ovarian hyperproduction of estrogen as a result of polycystic ovary syndrome or a theca cell tumor). Histologically, three forms of endometrial hyperplasia are recognized:

   1. **Simple hyperplasia** is characterized by cystic, dilated glands (**"Swiss cheese" appearance**).

   2. **Complex hyperplasia** is characterized by crowded glands that are hypercellular but show no nuclear atypia.

   3. **Complex hyperplasia with atypia** is characterized by irregularly shaped glands showing nuclear atypia.

B. **Endometriosis** is the appearance of foci of endometrial tissue outside the uterus (e.g., on the ovaries, uterine ligaments, or pelvic peritoneum). The ectopic endometrial tissue shows cyclic changes synchronous with those of the endometrium.

   1. **Pathologic findings**
      a. The serosal surfaces of the pelvic organs are sprinkled with **red, bluish,** or **yellow punctate lesions.** Bluish lesions are referred to as **"gunpowder mark" lesions.**
      b. The ectopic endometrial tissue consists of hemorrhagic endometrial stroma and glands. Blood-filled cysts (**"chocolate cysts"**) measuring 3–5 centimeters and larger may be found on the ovaries.

   2. **Clinical findings.** Cyclic enlargement and interstitial bleeding causes **pelvic pain,** which is most pronounced at the time of menstruation. Oral contraceptives suppress cyclic changes and provide relief.

   3. **Complications.** Infertility is the most common complication, although it is not known why it occurs. Fibrosis and adhesions also occur.

C. **Ovarian cysts** are non-neoplastic fluid-filled cavities that may be solitary or multiple.

   1. Cyst formation is related to subclinical hormonal disturbances.

   2. The cysts are classified as follicular, theca-luteal, or luteal.

D. **Polycystic ovary syndrome.** Biochemically, polycystic ovary syndrome is characterized by an excess of androgens and luteinizing hormone (LH), and a deficit of follicle-stimulating hormone (FSH).

   1. **Pathologic findings** include bilateral ovarian enlargement, cortical fibrosis, and multiple follicular cysts.

   2. **Clinical findings** may include amenorrhea, irregular ovulation, virilization, and infertility.

III. NEOPLASMS OF THE FEMALE REPRODUCTIVE TRACT. Although benign tumors of the female reproductive tract are more common than malignant tumors, malignant tumors of the reproductive tract account for 15% of all malignancies in women.

A. **Vulvar carcinoma,** seen primarily in elderly women, accounts for 3% of genital cancers. Most malignant vulvar tumors (95%) are **squamous cell carcinomas.** Invasive cancer is preceded by vulvar intraepithelial neoplasia (VIN), which is graded from I to III in a manner similar to that used for preinvasive carcinoma of the cervix (see II C 2).

B. Vaginal carcinoma

    1. **Vaginal squamous cell carcinoma** accounts for only 1% of all genital cancers. Patients with vaginal carcinoma may also have vulvar or cervical cancer, suggesting a common cause (e.g., HPV infection).

    2. **Vaginal clear cell adenocarcinoma** is seen in young women who were exposed to diethylstilbestrol (DES) during fetal development.

> **Vaginal clear cell adenocarcinoma is an example of transplacental carcinogenesis in humans.**

C. **Cervical carcinoma** accounts for 20% of gynecologic cancers.

    1. **Risk factors** for the development of cervical carcinoma include **HPV infection, the early onset of sexual activity,** and **promiscuity.**

    2. **Pathologic findings.** Most tumors originate from the transitional zone and are **squamous cell carcinomas.** Invasive cervical carcinoma is preceded by **cervical intraepithelial neoplasia (CIN),** a curable condition. CIN I **(mild dysplasia)** shows disorderly maturation limited to the basal and parabasal layers, whereas CIN III shows atypical cells through the entire thickness of the epithelium **(carcinoma *in situ*).**

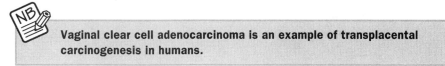

> **Widespread use of the Papanicolaou smear, which is used to detect CIN, has markedly decreased the incidence of invasive cervical cancer in the United States.**

    3. **Prognosis.** Tumor stage is the primary determinant of prognosis. CIN is labeled as stage 0, whereas invasive cancer is staged I–IV, depending on the extent of tumor spread.

D. **Uterine tumors.** The uterus is the most common site of tumors in the female reproductive system.

    1. **Endometrial carcinoma,** the most common gynecologic malignancy, accounts for 50% of all gynecologic cancers.

        a. **Risk factors** are **nulliparity, obesity, diabetes mellitus,** and **hyperestrinism.**

        b. **Pathologic findings.** More than 95% of endometrial cancers are **adenocarcinomas.** Other endometrial malignancies, such as endometrial stromal sarcoma (composed of stromal cells) or mixed mullerian tumors (composed of glandular and stromal malignant cells), are rare.

> **In women with vaginal bleeding or "spotting," endometrial biopsy can allow early detection of endometrial carcinoma.**

    2. **Myometrial tumors** are classified as leiomyomas or leiomyosarcomas.

        a. **Leiomyomas,** which are benign, account for 98% of all myometrial tumors, and are often multiple. Leiomyomas are classified as **submucosal, intramural,** or **subserosal** (Figure 14-2).

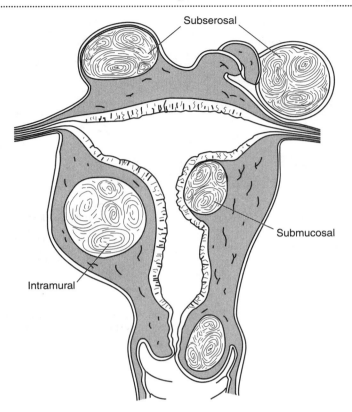

Figure 14-2. Leiomyomas may be classified as subserosal, intramural, or submucosal. Subserosal and submucosal tumors may be pedunculated; pedunculated subserosal leiomyomas protrude from the uterine surface, and pedunculated submucosal leiomyomas protrude into the uterine cavity. Symptoms depend on the location of the tumor: subserosal and intramural tumors produce a "mass effect" (e.g., symptoms related to compression of adjacent organs), and submucosal tumors may cause bleeding, dysmenorrhea, and infertility owing to impeded implantation.

       b. **Leiomyosarcomas,** rare malignant tumors that enlarge the uterus, may metastasize hematogenously to distant sites.

   E. **Ovarian tumors** (Figure 14-3) account for 6% of all neoplasms in women; malignant ovarian tumors are the fifth most common type of cancer in women.

      1. **Primary ovarian tumors** originate from four cell types (surface epithelial cells, germ cells, sex cord cells, and nonspecific stromal cells).

       a. **Surface epithelial cell tumors**

         (1) **Serous** and **mucinous tumors** are cystic; their cysts contain either serous fluid or mucus, respectively. Serous tumors are more often malignant and more often bilateral than mucinous tumors.

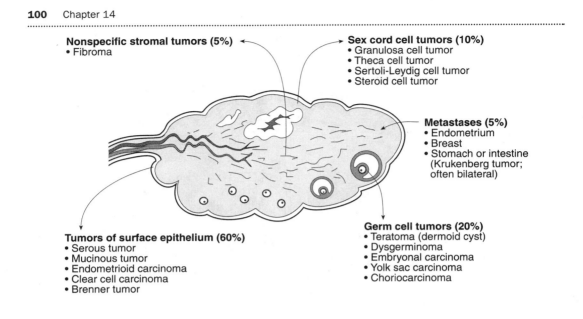

Figure 14-3.   Sources of ovarian tumors. Primary ovarian tumors can originate from surface epithelial cells, germ cells, sex cord cells, and nonspecific stroma. Sources of metastases to the ovary include the breast, uterus, and gastrointestinal tract.

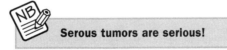

Serous tumors are serious!

> **(2)** **Endometrioid carcinomas** and **clear cell carcinomas** are solid malignant tumors.
>
> **(3)** **Brenner tumors** are benign, solid tumors composed of nests of transitional epithelium.

b. **Germ cell tumors** include teratomas (dermoid cysts), dysgerminomas, embryonal carcinomas, yolk sac carcinomas, and choriocarcinomas. Teratomas, which are benign, are the most common ovarian tumor in women younger than 25 years. All other ovarian germ cell tumors are malignant.

c. **Sex cord cell tumors** are rare tumors with a peak incidence in women between the ages of 25 and 45 years.

> **(1)** **Theca cell tumors,** which are benign, and **granulosa cell tumors,** which are low-grade malignancies, secrete estrogens.
>
> **(2)** **Sertoli-Leydig cell tumors,** which may be benign or malignant, secrete androgens.
>
> **(3)** **Steroid cell tumors,** which may be benign or malignant, originate from hilar cells and secrete androgens.

d. **Nonspecific stromal tumors.** Fibroma is the most common tumor of nonspecific ovarian stroma. This hormonally inactive tumor presents as a firm ("fibrotic") mass that expands or completely replaces the ovary. Ovarian fibromas may be associated with pleural effusion (Meigs syndrome).

> **In addition to involving the pelvic and abdominal lymph nodes, ovarian cancers tend to spread into the peritoneal cavity. Peritoneal seeding leads to the formation of malignant ascites. Mucinous adenocarcinomas secrete mucus that fills the peritoneal cavity (pseudomyxoma peritonei).**

2. **Metastases to the ovaries.** Most often, the primary tumor is endometrial adenocarcinoma, but metastases may also occur from the breast or gastrointestinal tract. Ovarian metastases from gastrointestinal adenocarcinomas are called **Krukenberg tumors.**

IV. DISORDERS ASSOCIATED WITH PREGNANCY

A. Ectopic pregnancy results from implantation of the conceptus outside of the uterine cavity.

1. The most common site for ectopic implantation is the **fallopian tube** (95% of cases); other sites include the **ovaries, cervix,** or **peritoneal surfaces.**

2. Ectopic pregnancies cannot be brought to term and usually result in spontaneous abortion or hemorrhage. Tubal pregnancy may cause rupture of the tube and hematoperitoneum.

B. Gestational trophoblastic disease (GTD) results from abnormal formation of the placenta and encompasses several entities, the most important of which are hydatidiform mole and choriocarcinoma. GTD is ten times more common in Southeast Asia (as compared with the United States, where it is rare).

1. **Hydatidiform mole** is characterized by marked swelling of the chorionic villi, associated with variable degrees of trophoblastic cell hyperplasia. If all of the villi are involved, the mole is **complete,** and if only some of the villi are involved, the mole is **partial.**
   a. **Pathogenesis.** Hydatidiform mole develops as a result of abnormal fertilization.
      (1) **Complete moles** have a 46,XX karyotype, which results from **androgenesis,** a process in which the fertilized ovum loses the maternal chromosomes but retains the paternal chromosomes.
      (2) **Incomplete moles** have a triploid karyotype (69,XXY or 69,XYY) and contain one female haploid set and two male haploid sets of chromosomes.
   b. **Clinical findings.** Hydatidiform moles produce excessive amounts of human chorionic gonadotropin (hCG) and cause enlargement of the uterus that is out of proportion with the duration of the pregnancy. No fetal movement is noticed.
   c. **Treatment.** Most moles abort spontaneously, but if they do not, then curettage and evacuation is curative.

> **2%–3% of complete moles tend to become invasive and recur after evacuation, possibly giving rise to choriocarcinoma.**

   2. **Choriocarcinoma** is a rare, malignant, highly invasive tumor with a tendency toward hematogenous metastases.
      a. **Pathogenesis.** In 50% of cases, choriocarcinoma is a complication of hydatidiform mole, in 25% of cases it follows abortion, and in 25% of cases, it occurs after a normal pregnancy.
      b. **Pathologic findings.** The tumor is composed of trophoblastic cells: **mononuclear cytotrophoblastic cells and multinuclear syncytiotrophoblastic cells.**
      c. **Clinical findings.** Choriocarcinomas produce large amounts of hCG.
      d. **Treatment.** Despite widespread metastases, a cure rate in excess of 75% has been achieved using chemotherapy regimens that contain **methotrexate.** Only when the tumor has metastasized to the brain is the prognosis poor.

   C. **Preeclampsia** is defined clinically as the triad of proteinuria, edema, and hypertension developing during the third trimester of pregnancy. Vigorous treatment with magnesium salts can prevent its progression to eclampsia, which is often lethal.

V. DISORDERS OF THE BREAST

   A. **Women.** Breasts are secondary sex organs that develop in response to estrogens and achieve full maturity only after pregnancy and lactation.

   1. **Mastitis** is inflammation of the breast.
      a. **Acute mastitis** is a bacterial infection that typically occurs during lactation. Incomplete evacuation of the milk and the minor skin trauma (fissures of the nipple) caused by suckling predispose to bacterial invasion.
      b. **Chronic mastitis (plasma cell mastitis, mammary duct ectasia)** is a disease of unknown etiology that affects perimenopausal women and produces nonspecific symptoms. Most importantly, it should be distinguished from carcinoma.

   2. **Fibrocystic change,** found in approximately 50% of women older than 40 years, is the most common histologic diagnosis on breast tissue biopsies. Gross and microscopic changes are related to the cumulative effects of cyclic hormonal changes, which affect the epithelium and stroma of the adult female breast.
      a. **Pathologic findings.** Fibrocystic change is characterized by **irregular ("beadlike") nodularity, lumps,** and **fibrotic thickening** of the breast parenchyma. It is typically bilateral.
      b. **Clinical findings** (e.g., breast pain) are more prominent prior to menstruation.

   3. **Benign breast tumors**
      a. **Fibroadenomas** are benign tumors characterized by proliferation of the ducts and intralobular stroma. Fibroadenomas are the most common tumor in young women, with a peak incidence in the 20- to 25-year age group.
      b. **Phyllodes tumors** are **giant fibroadenomas.** Phyllodes tumors are usually benign but in some cases, they are low-grade malignancies.

   4. **Carcinoma of the breast** is the most common malignancy among women—one of every 12 women can expect to develop breast cancer during her lifetime, and breast cancer accounts for 20% of cancer deaths in the United States. Breast carcinoma has a tendency to metastasize to local lymph nodes, most often those located in the axilla or along the internal mammary artery. Distant hematogenous metastases are found in the lungs, liver, brain, adrenal glands, and ovaries.
      a. **Risk factors.** The most important risk factors for the development of breast cancer are summarized in Table 14-1.
      b. **Types of breast cancer**
         (1) **Infiltrating ductal carcinoma** accounts for 70% of cases of breast cancer. Most tumors originate in the outer upper quadrant and, at the time of di-

Table 14-1
Risk Factors for Breast Cancer

Sex	Female > male = 100:1
Race	Caucasians > Asians = 5:1
Age	50 years > 30 years = 10:1
Family history	Positive > negative = 10:1
Obstetric history	Nulliparous > multiparous
	Late age at first pregnancy > early pregnancy
	No breast feeding > breast feeding
Other pathology	Proliferative fibrocystic disease
	Cancer of the contralateral breast
	Ovarian cancer

Reprinted with permission from Damjanov I, Conran PH, Goldblatt PJ: *Rypins' Intensive Reviews: Pathology.* Philadelphia, Lippincott-Raven, 1998, p 229.

agnosis, measure 2–4 centimeters in diameter and are hard (scirrhous). By mammography, most tumors appear dense and show focal calcification.

> **Paget disease is a form of invasive breast cancer that originates in the ducts and spreads intraductally to invade the skin of the nipple. It is an invasive cancer and thus has an unfavorable prognosis. Clinically, Paget disease presents as eczema of the nipple.**

(2) **Lobular carcinoma** is also a scirrhous carcinoma, clinically indistinguishable from infiltrating ductal carcinoma. Histologically, the lobular carcinoma cells are smaller and tend to infiltrate the connective tissue as single cell columns **("Indian file" patterns).** Lobular carcinoma is bilateral in 30% of cases.

(3) **Medullary, mucinous,** and **tubular carcinomas** are rare forms of breast cancer. These tumors are associated with a better prognosis than infiltrating ductal and lobular carcinomas.

  c. **Clinical findings.** Symptoms of breast carcinoma are nonspecific.

    (1) **Small parenchymal nodules** may be detected on palpation.

    (2) **Nipple retraction, nipple discharge,** and **breast inflammation** are rare but important signs.

    (3) **Lymph node enlargement** (as a result of metastases) is common. It also may be the first sign of disease, leading to recognition of some small breast tumors.

    (4) **Paraneoplastic findings** (e.g., hypercalcemia) are found in advanced disease.

  d. **Prognosis.** The prognosis depends on the stage of the tumor, the histologic type, and the presence or absence of estrogen receptors.

B. **Men.** Male breasts are underdeveloped and nonfunctioning; therefore, breast diseases are less common in men than in women.

  1. **Gynecomastia** is enlargement of the male breast, usually in response to relative hyperestrinism.

    a. High serum estrogen concentrations are seen in patients with **estrogen-secreting tumors of the testis** or the **adrenal gland.**

    b. Relatively mild elevations of serum estrogen levels may be related to **drugs** or **metabolic disorders** (e.g., cirrhosis).

2. Carcinoma of the male breast is 100 times less common than carcinoma of the female breast. Histologically, it is most often of the infiltrating duct type.

15

Pathology of the Endocrine System

I. DISORDERS OF THE ANTERIOR PITUITARY GLAND. Dysfunction of the anterior pituitary gland affects the thyroid gland, the adrenal cortex, and the gonads.

A. Hyperpituitarism is most often caused by **benign tumors** (Table 15-1), which are classified as microadenomas (< 1 cm in diameter) or macroadenomas (≥ 1 cm in diameter).

> **All anterior pituitary tumors may expand the sella turcica, compress the optic chiasm (leading to bitemporal hemianopsia), or compress the normal gland (leading to hormonal deficiencies).**

B. Hypopituitarism. Loss of 75% of the anterior pituitary gland leads to hypopituitarism, as does destruction of the hypothalamus or the hypothalamic–pituitary tract (pituitary stalk). Causes of hypopituitarism include:

1. Tumors
   a. Nonfunctioning pituitary adenoma
   b. **Craniopharyngioma,** a benign tumor originating from remnants of the Rathke pouch and usually located in or above the sella turcica
   c. **Glioma,** which can destroy the hypothalamic centers on the hypothalamic-pituitary tract

2. **Trauma** (e.g., head injury, surgery) may damage the hypothalamic–pituitary tract.

3. **Sheehan syndrome** (postpartum ischemic pituitary necrosis) is a rare cause of hypopituitarism in women.

II. DISORDERS OF THE POSTERIOR PITUITARY GLAND. The posterior pituitary gland releases antidiuretic hormone (ADH, vasopressin) and oxytocin. These hormones are synthesized in the supraoptic and paraventricular nuclei of the hypothalamus.

A. Diabetes insipidus is caused by destruction of the hypothalamus or posterior pituitary gland. ADH deficiency leads to uncontrollable loss of water in the urine and concentration of sodium in the remaining reduced fluid volume (hypernatremia).

B. Syndrome of inappropriate ADH secretion (SIADH). An excess of ADH leads to water retention and dilutional hyponatremia. Causes of SIADH include:

1. **Chronic lung disease,** such as **small cell carcinoma of the lung** (the most common cause) or **tuberculosis**

Table 15-1
Pituitary Adenomas

Tumor	Incidence	Hormone Secreted in Excess*	Clinical Manifestations
Prolactinoma	30%	Prolactin	Amenorrhea–galactorrhea syndrome (in women); hypotension and loss of libido (in men)
Corticotroph adenoma	15%	ACTH	Cushing disease
Gonadotroph adenoma	10%	LH, FSH	Menstrual disturbances (in women); loss of libido (in men)
Thyrotroph adenoma	10%	TSH	Hyperthyroidism (high serum TSH, T_3, and T_4 levels)
Somatotroph adenoma	5%	Growth hormone	Gigantism (in prepubertal children); acromegaly (in adults)

ACTH = adrenocorticotropic hormone; FSH = follicle-stimulating hormone; LH = luteinizing hormone; T_3 = triiodothyronine; T_4 = thyroxine; TSH = thyroid-stimulating hormone.
*Thirty percent of pituitary adenomas are nonfunctioning.

2. Drugs, such as certain **psychotropic agents, diuretics,** and **cytostatic agents**

3. Hypothalamic hyperfunction (the rarest cause)

III. DISORDERS OF THE THYROID GLAND cause metabolic disorders related to an excess or deficiency of thyroid hormones.

    A. Hyperthyroidism presents with signs of hypermetabolism (Figure 15-1).

        1. Graves disease, an autoimmune disease mediated by antibodies to thyroid-stimulating hormone (TSH) receptors, is the most common cause of hyperthyroidism. Antibodies bound to TSH receptors stimulate thyroid cells to synthesize thyroxine (T_4).

            a. Epidemiology. Women are affected five times more often than men. The peak incidence is in the 20- to 40-year age group.

            b. Pathologic findings include hyperplastic follicular epithelium, "scalloping" where the colloid meets the follicular epithelium (owing to accelerated resorption of colloid), and lymphoid infiltrates.

            c. Clinical findings. Graves disease is the prototypical example of hyperthyroidism (see Figure 15-1).

        2. Toxic thyroid adenoma is a solitary hyperfunctioning benign tumor of the follicular epithelium.

        3. Toxic multinodular goiter is a hormonally active form of thyroid hyperplasia.

        4. TSH-secreting pituitary adenoma is a rare cause of hyperthyroidism.

    B. Hypothyroidism presents with signs of hypometabolism (Figure 15-2).

        1. Congenital hypothyroidism results from agenesis of the thyroid or a deficiency of the enzymes involved in T_4 synthesis. Clinical findings include:

            a. Dwarfism (owing to retarded bone growth)

            b. Mental retardation (historically often referred to as "cretinism")

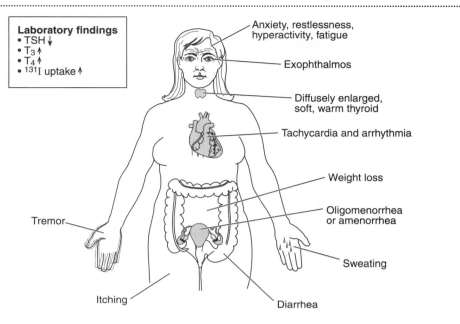

Figure 15-1.   Clinical features of hyperthyroidism. In all hyperthyroid conditions, radioactive iodine (^{131}I) accumulates in the lesion, registering as either diffuse uptake or a solitary "hot nodule" on ^{131}I isotope scans. T_3 = triiodothyronine; T_4 = thyroxine; TSH = thyroid-stimulating hormone.

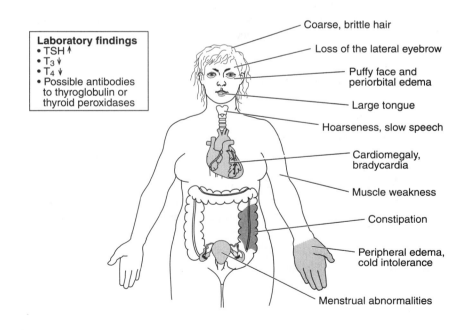

Figure 15-2.   Clinical features of hypothyroidism. T_3 = triiodothyronine; T_4 = thyroxine; TSH = thyroid-stimulating hormone.

    c. Myxedema (i.e., dry, waxy swelling of the skin of the extremities and face)

    d. **Low serum triiodothyronine (T_3) and T_4 levels** with compensatory **high serum TSH levels**

2. **Endemic iodine deficiency,** although absent in the United States, is still prevalent in the mountainous regions of South America and Southeast Asia. In children, endemic iodine deficiency leads to **cretinism** (i.e., severe mental retardation, short stature, coarse facial features, a protruding tongue, and umbilical hernia), whereas in adults, it leads to **nodular goiter** (i.e., enlargement of the thyroid gland).

3. Thyroiditis

    a. **Hashimoto thyroiditis,** an autoimmune disease, is the most common cause of hypothyroidism in the United States. Women are affected ten times more often than men.

        (1) **Pathologic findings.** Microscopic infiltration of the thyroid with lymphocytes leads to destruction of normal follicles. The remaining follicles show oncocytic change (i.e., their cytoplasm is pink owing to an increased number of mitochondria).

        (2) **Clinical findings** include goiter and, in advanced cases, hypothyroidism. Serum TSH levels are high, and serum T_3 and T_4 levels are low. Antibodies to thyroglobulin are present in the serum, but not are not diagnostic.

    b. **Rare forms of thyroiditis** include **subacute thyroiditis** (also known as **granulomatous thyroiditis** or **deQuervain thyroiditis),** which is probably caused by viral infection, and **Riedel thyroiditis,** a fibrosing disease of unknown etiology.

> **Lymphocytic thyroiditis, the most common form of thyroid inflammation of unknown etiology, does not cause functional disturbances (i.e., patients are euthyroid).**

C. **Thyroid neoplasms** are most often benign tumors or low-grade malignancies. Women are affected more often than men.

1. **Thyroid adenoma,** the most common thyroid neoplasm, is a benign tumor of the follicular epithelium that usually presents as a nonfunctioning ("cold") nodule.

2. **Thyroid carcinomas** are summarized in Table 15-2.

> **Tumors of the thyroid must be distinguished from nodular goiter, the most common cause of thyroid enlargement. In most instances in the United States, the cause of nodular goiter is not known.**

IV. **DISORDERS OF THE PARATHYROID GLAND** cause disturbances in the homeostasis of body calcium and phosphate.

    A. Hyperparathyroidism

        1. Causes

            a. **Primary hyperparathyroidism** is characterized by the spontaneous hypersecretion of parathyroid hormone (PTH).

Table 15-2
Malignant Tumors of the Thyroid Gland

Tumor	Incidence*	Pathologic Findings	Prognosis
Papillary carcinoma	70%	Papillae are lined by cuboidal cells with clear nuclei ("Orphan Annie" nuclei); psammoma bodies	Low-grade malignancy; survival rate is 85% at 20 years, despite tendency for early metastasis to ipsilateral cervical lymph nodes
Follicular carcinoma	20%	Composed of follicular cells, which may form colloid and concentrate radioactive iodine	Aggressive; the prognosis depends on the cellular degree of differentiation and the tumor stage (e.g., capsule involvement, presence of distant metastases)
Medullary carcinoma[†]	5%	Amyloid deposits in the tumor stroma; elevated serum levels of calcitonin and possibly other polypeptide hormones (e.g., VIP)	Aggressive; survival rate is 50% at 5 years; patients with familial medullary carcinoma generally have a better prognosis
Undifferentiated carcinoma	1%	Pleomorphic cells arranged in solid sheets	Highly malignant tumor exhibiting rapid growth and metastasis; most patients die within 1 year

VIP = vasoactive intestinal peptide.
*Among malignant tumors.
[†]This aggressive tumor of C cells may be sporadic (80% of cases) or familial. Familial medullary carcinoma may be a part of multiple endocrine neoplasia (MEN), types 2a and 2b, or it may occur outside of these syndromes.

        (1) A **solitary parathyroid adenoma** is responsible for primary hyperparathyroidism in 80% of patients.

        (2) **Primary hyperplasia** of all four parathyroid glands is responsible for hyperparathyroidism in 15% of patients.

        (3) **Parathyroid carcinoma** causes primary hyperparathyroidism in 5% of patients. This tumor is characterized by invasive growth and metastases.

    b. **Secondary hyperparathyroidism.** Diffuse enlargement of all four parathyroid glands is seen in response to hypocalcemia, such as occurs in **end-stage renal disease, malabsorption syndromes,** or **vitamin D deficiency.**

    c. **Tertiary hyperparathyroidism,** characterized by diffuse enlargement of all four parathyroid glands and the autonomous hypersecretion of PTH, follows secondary hyperparathyroidism and persists even after the cause of parathyroid hyperplasia has been eliminated (e.g., following a renal transplant in a patient with end-stage renal disease).

2. Clinical findings are the same for all forms of hyperparathyroidism:

    a. **Serum calcium** and **PTH levels** are **elevated,** but the phosphate concentration is variable, depending on the cause of the hyperparathyroidism.

In most instances, the hypercalcemia is mild (i.e., asymptomatic) and discovered during routine laboratory testing.

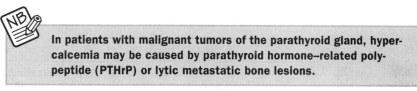

In patients with malignant tumors of the parathyroid gland, hypercalcemia may be caused by parathyroid hormone–related polypeptide (PTHrP) or lytic metastatic bone lesions.

b. Demineralization of the bones results in **bone softening** and **painful fractures** (**osteitis cystica fibrosa** in primary hyperparathyroidism, **renal osteodystrophy** in secondary hyperparathyroidism).

c. Hypercalciuria predisposes to **urinary calculi.**

d. Constipation, peptic ulcers, pancreatitis, and biliary stones are sources of **abdominal pain.**

e. Mental symptoms include **depression** and **lethargy.**

f. **Cardiac arrhythmias** may be seen.

Think "painful bones, kidney stones, belly groans, and mental moans" to remember the major clinical manifestations of hyperparathyroidism.

B. **Hypoparathyroidism** is much less common than hyperparathyroidism.

1. Causes
  a. **Parathyroid gland aplasia** (e.g., DiGeorge syndrome)
  b. **Surgical removal** (usually accidental, during thyroid or neck surgery)
  c. **Autoimmune** or **familial pluriglandular endocrine insufficiency**

2. Clinical findings
  a. Serum calcium levels are **decreased,** while **serum phosphate levels** are **increased.**
  b. **Neuromuscular hyperexcitability** may be manifested as **carpopedal spasm, laryngospasm, Chvostek sign** (i.e., spasm of the facial muscles), or **Trousseau phenomenon** (i.e., muscles spasms provoked by the application of pressure to the nerves that supply them).
  c. **Calcifications in the basal ganglia** and **cataracts** may be seen.
  d. **Bone changes** vary from **osteosclerosis** to **osteomalacia.**
  e. **Seizures, cardiac arrest,** or both may be seen in severe cases.

V. DISORDERS OF THE ADRENAL CORTEX are associated with complex disorders involving the intermediate metabolism of carbohydrates and lipids. In addition, sodium and potassium imbalances are seen.

A. Adrenocortical hyperfunction

  1. **Hyperaldosteronism (Conn syndrome)** is caused by **adenomas** composed of cells resembling the mineralocorticoid-secreting cells of the zona glomerulosa. Retention of salt and water leads to hypertension, and potassium loss leads to muscle weakness.

Primary hyperaldosteronism must be distinguished from secondary hyperaldosteronism, which is caused by renin release and is seen in patients with renal disease.

2. Hypercortisolism (Cushing syndrome)

   a. **Causes.** The most common cause of hypercortisolism is the **administration of exogenous steroids.** Other, endogenous, causes include:

   (1) **Primary adrenocortical hyperplasia** or **neoplasia**

   (2) **Adrenocorticotropic hormone (ACTH)–secreting pituitary adenomas** (Cushing disease)

   (3) **ACTH-secreting nonendocrine neoplasms** (e.g., small cell lung carcinoma)

   b. **Clinical findings** are shown in Figure 15-3.

3. Androgen hypersecretion (adrenogenital syndrome)

   a. **Causes** include **adrenocortical tumors** composed of cells resembling those of the zona reticularis and **congenital adrenogenital syndrome** (caused by 21-hydroxylase deficiency).

   b. **Clinical findings** are summarized in Table 15-3.

B. Adrenocortical hypofunction

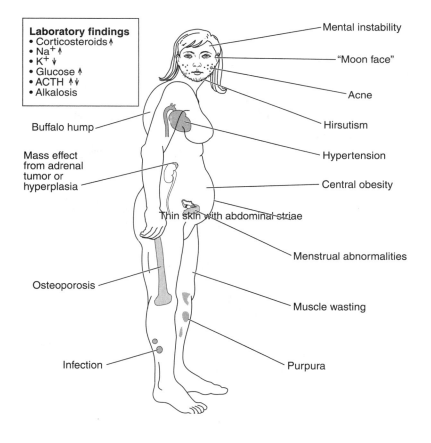

Laboratory findings
- Corticosteroids ↑
- Na$^+$ ↑
- K$^+$ ↓
- Glucose ↑
- ACTH ↑↓
- Alkalosis

Buffalo hump

Mass effect from adrenal tumor or hyperplasia

Osteoporosis

Infection

Mental instability

"Moon face"

Acne

Hirsutism

Hypertension

Central obesity

Thin skin with abdominal striae

Menstrual abnormalities

Muscle wasting

Purpura

Figure 15-3. Clinical features of hypercortisolism. When hypercortisolism results from exogenous administration of steroids or primary adrenal disease, the serum cortisol levels are high, but the serum adrenocorticotropic hormone (*ACTH*) levels are low. This is in contrast to hypercortisolism resulting from pituitary adenomas or nonendocrine neoplasms, in which both serum cortisol and ACTH levels are elevated. ACTH stimulates melanocytes causing hyperpigmentation of skin, which is not seen in primary adrenal disease. K^+ = potassium; Na^+ = sodium.

1. Acute adrenocortical insufficiency (Waterhouse-Friderichsen syndrome) is caused by meningococcal septicemia.

2. Chronic adrenocortical insufficiency (Addison disease)
   a. Causes include **autoimmune adrenalitis,** (65% of cases), **infections** (e.g.,

Table 15-3
Clinical Findings in Adrenogenital Syndromes

Patient	Findings
Prepubertal female	Virilization of external genitalia, which may appear ambiguous
Postpubertal female	Clitoromegaly, male-type hirsutism, deepening of the voice, menstrual irregularities
Prepubertal male	Premature puberty
Postpubertal male	Asymptomatic or paradoxical oligospermia

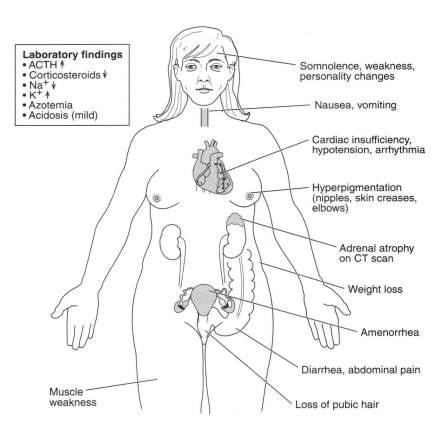

Figure 15-4. Clinical features of chronic adrenal insufficiency (Addison disease). Many of the signs and symptoms derive from disturbances of the sodium–potassium balance and disturbances in the metabolism of glucose and lipids. *ACTH* = adrenocorticotropic hormone; *CT* = computed tomography; K^+ = potassium; Na^+ = sodium.

AIDS, histoplasmosis, tuberculosis), and **metastatic tumors** (especially from the lung and breast).

  b. **Clinical findings** are shown in Figure 15-4.

VI. DISORDERS OF THE ADRENAL MEDULLA. Tumors (the only significant lesion of the adrenal medulla) cause hypertension and other metabolic disturbances as a result of hypersecretion of catecholamines.

  A. **Neuroblastoma,** a tumor composed of malignant neuroblasts similar to the neural crest precursors of adrenal medullary cells, is seen in children younger than 5 years. Although most neuroblastomas arise from the adrenal glands, similar tumors can originate from the sympathetic ganglia and (rarely) from the central nervous system (CNS).

   1. **Pathologic findings.** The tumor cells are small, round, and stain blue because they contain very little cytoplasm.

   2. **Clinical findings.** The tumor cells secrete catecholamines [e.g., vanillylmandelic acid (VMA)], leading hypertension and elevated urine levels of these substances.

   3. **Prognosis.** The rapidly proliferating cells respond well to chemotherapy; the 5-year survival rate is 80%.

  B. **Pheochromocytoma** is a tumor composed of cells resembling the normal cells of the adrenal medulla. Symptoms include bouts of paroxysmal hypertension, headaches, sweating, tachycardia, and nervousness.

> **When thinking about pheochromocytoma, remember the "rule of 90%":**
> **90% are benign; 10% are malignant.**
> **90% secrete adrenalin or noradrenalin; 10% are afunctional.**
> **90% are solitary; 10% are bilateral.**
> **90% occur in the adrenals; 10% are extraadrenal.**
> **90% are sporadic; 10% are familial (a component of MEN type 2).**

16

Pathology of the Skin

I. INTRODUCTION. Table 16-1 summarizes the most common morphologic types of skin lesions.

II. INFECTIOUS DISORDERS

   A. Bacterial infections

      1. **Acute bacterial infections** are usually caused by pus-forming *Staphylococcus* and *Streptococcus* species.

         a. **Impetigo** is a superficial skin infection most often seen in children. Patients present with groups of small, oozing, crust-covered pustules, usually on the face or hands.

         b. **Furuncles** are abscesses within the confines of hair follicles. **Carbuncles** (boils) are confluent furuncles.

         c. **Suppurative hidradenitis** is an infection of the sweat glands, most often in the groin or axilla.

         d. **Erysipelas** is infection of the dermis and subcutis of the hands or feet. Patients present with swelling and redness of the overlying epidermis and linear centrifugal extension through the lymphatics.

         e. **Cellulitis** is an infection of the deep subcutis that extends into adjacent soft tissues.

      2. Chronic bacterial infections

         a. **Syphilis**

            (1) **Condylomata lata** (papules or plaques, typically located in intertriginous areas) may be a feature of **secondary syphilis.**

            (2) **Gummas** (dermal granulomas with central necrosis and a peripheral plasma cell infiltrate) may be seen in **tertiary syphilis.**

         b. **Leprosy** is characterized by induration of the skin owing to dermal infiltrates of macrophages and granuloma formation.

         c. **Acne vulgaris** is infection of the pilosebaceous units of the face, back, and upper chest by *Propionibacterium acnes*, a bacterium that thrives in stagnant sebum. Teenagers are affected most often; hormonal and genetic factors are thought to play a role.

   B. Viral infections

      1. Childhood exanthems

         a. **Measles (rubeola)** is a maculopapular rash that begins on the face and behind the ears and spreads to the trunk.

Table 16-1
Morphology of Skin Lesions

Lesion	Illustration	Description	Example
Macule	Epidermis — Dermis —	Flat lesion of a different color than normal skin	Freckle
Papule		Slightly elevated lesion	Eczema
Plaque		Papule larger than 5 mm in diameter	Psoriasis
Nodule, tumor		Defined, often protruding mass	Malignant melanoma
Vesicle, bulla	Fluid —	Fluid-filled blister (vesicles are small and bullae are large)	Herpes, burn injury
Pustule		Pus-filled blister	Folliculitis
Ulcer	Exposed dermis	Defect in the epidermis	Stasis ulcer on legs

(continued)

Table 16-1—*Continued*
Morphology of Skin Lesions

Lesion	Illustration	Description	Example
Crust (scab)		A covering formed of coagulated blood over a skin defect	Healing wound
Scale		Layers of keratin that are easily removed by scratching	Chronic dermatitis

b. Varicella (chicken pox) is characterized by the appearance of vesicles on the face, scalp, and trunk, extending later to the arms and legs.

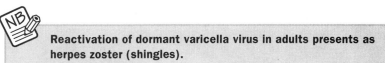

Reactivation of dormant varicella virus in adults presents as herpes zoster (shingles).

2. Herpes simplex virus (HSV) infections present as small groups of vesicles.
  a. HSV-1 causes herpes labialis (i.e., a "cold sore").
  b. HSV-2 causes genital herpes.
  c. HSV-8 causes Kaposi sarcoma.

3. Human papilloma virus (HPV) infection causes warts.
  a. Verruca vulgaris is the common wart, seen most often on the arms and legs.
  b. Plantar warts are flat warts on the soles of the feet.
  c. Condylomata acuminata are large genital warts.

C. Fungal infections
  1. Superficial fungal infections are caused by dermatophytes (e.g., *Trichophyton, Epidermophyton,* or *Microsporum* species).
    a. Tinea capitis is characterized by patches of hair loss from the scalp.
    b. Tinea cruris ("jock itch"). Patients present with itchy scales and patches in the groin.
    c. Tinea corporis ("ringworm"). Lesions, usually located on the trunk, are pale patches with raised margins.
    d. Tinea pedis ("athletes foot") is characterized by scales and rhagades (i.e., fissures in the skin) between the toes.
  2. Deep fungal infections are caused by *Blastomyces* species and related fungi. These infections typically occur in the tropics and are rare in the United States. They are

characterized by a granulomatous reaction accompanied by suppuration ("deep boils"), tissue destruction, and disfigurement.

D. Parasitic infections. Scabies is a chronic skin infection caused by *Sarcoptes scabiei*, a mite that invades the epidermis. Patients present with migratory maculopapular rashes.

III. IMMUNE-MEDIATED DISORDERS. All four types of hypersensitivity reactions may affect the skin (Figure 16-1).

A. Type I (anaphylactic) reactions. Atopic dermatitis is an allergic reaction to food or environmental antigens, most commonly seen in infants and children. Clinical features of atopic dermatitis include **urticaria** (local edema and wheal formation) and **pruritus,** which provokes scratching. Eczema (chronic dermatitis) may result from scratching and secondary infection.

B. Type II (antibody-mediated) reactions

1. Pemphigus vulgaris is characterized by widespread **intraepidermal blisters** resulting from loss of normal intracellular attachments in the epidermis. Loss of the epidermis predisposes to infection, which accounts for the high mortality rate associated with this condition. Immunofluorescence microscopy shows linear deposits of IgG along the surface of keratinocytes.

2. Bullous pemphigoid is characterized by **subepidermal blisters.** Clinically, lesions are noted on the inner thighs, the flexor surfaces of the arms, or the oral mucosa. Immunofluorescence microscopy shows linear deposits of IgG along the epidermal–dermal basement membrane.

C. Type III (immune complex–mediated) reactions

1. Systemic lupus erythematosus (SLE). The classic facial "butterfly" rash and the scaly, erythematous plaques that develop on sun-exposed areas in some patients with SLE are caused by the deposition of circulating immune complexes at the epidermal–dermal junction. Immunofluorescence microscopy reveals granular deposits of IgG and complement along the epidermal–dermal junction (this is known as a **"positive lupus band test").**

2. Discoid lupus erythematosus, a form of lupus that is limited to the skin, is characterized by discoid, scaling plaques **(hyperkeratosis).** Lymphocytic infiltrates are seen around the dermal vessels and skin appendages (i.e., apocrine units). As in SLE, the lupus band test is positive.

D. Type IV (cell-mediated) reactions are mediated by T cells. **Sarcoidosis** and **contact dermatitis** (e.g., latex allergy, "poison ivy") are type IV hypersensitivity reactions.

IV. SKIN DISORDERS OF UNKNOWN ETIOLOGY

A. Psoriasis is a chronic disease that presents as recurrent eruptions of red or silvery papules, plaques, and scales. Lesions are most common on the elbows, knees, buttocks, and scalp. Microscopic changes include epidermal hyperplasia (i.e., acanthosis), parakeratosis (i.e., retention of nuclei in keratinized surface cells), and elongation of the dermal papillae.

> *NB*
>
> **Blood vessels within the dermal papillae bleed when the plaque is scraped away (Auspitz sign).**

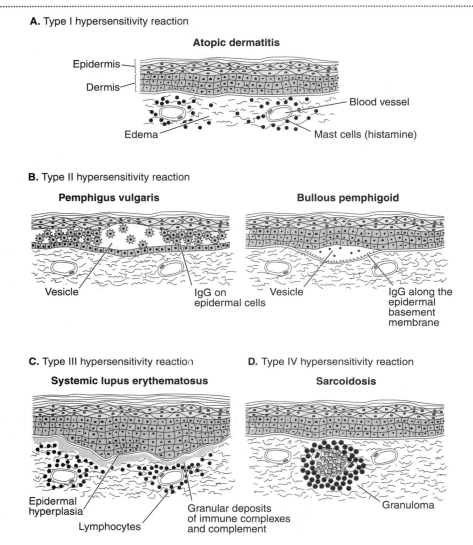

A. Type I hypersensitivity reaction

Atopic dermatitis

Epidermis
Dermis
Blood vessel
Edema
Mast cells (histamine)

B. Type II hypersensitivity reaction

Pemphigus vulgaris

Vesicle
IgG on epidermal cells

Bullous pemphigoid

Vesicle
IgG along the epidermal basement membrane

C. Type III hypersensitivity reaction

Systemic lupus erythematosus

Epidermal hyperplasia
Lymphocytes
Granular deposits of immune complexes and complement

D. Type IV hypersensitivity reaction

Sarcoidosis

Granuloma

Figure 16-1. Immune-mediated skin disorders. (A) Atopic dermatitis, a type I hypersensitivity reaction, is mediated by IgE antibodies, which are bound to the surfaces of mast cells in the dermis. The antigen-antibody reaction causes the mast cells to release histamine and other vasoactive substances, leading to edema of the dermis and epidermis. (B) Pemphigus vulgaris is mediated by IgG antibodies to a plasma membrane protein on the keratinocytes in the epidermis. Acantholysis (i.e., separation of the keratinocytes from one another) leads to the formation of intraepidermal vesicles and bullae, which are prone to rupture. Bullous pemphigoid is mediated by IgG antibodies against the hemidesmosome proteins, which anchor the basal cells of the epidermis to the epidermal basement membrane. Subepidermal vesicles and bullae form following detachment of the epidermis from the epidermal basement membrane. The vesicles and bullae of bullous pemphigoid do not rupture as easily as those of pemphigus vulgaris. (C) In systemic lupus erythematosus (SLE), the "butterfly" rash is caused by the deposition of circulating immune complexes at the junction of the epidermis and dermis. Immune complex deposition activates complement, which, in addition to being cytotoxic to keratinocytes, is chemotactic, attracting inflammatory cells to the dermis. (D) Sarcoidosis, a systemic granulomatous reaction of unknown etiology, is characterized by the formation of noncaseating granulomas in the dermis.

B. Lichen planus is a self-limited eruption of pruritic red papules on the flexor surfaces of the extremities, the genitals, and the oral mucosa. Microscopic examination reveals infiltrates of T lymphocytes in the upper dermis and epidermis.

V. NEOPLASTIC DISORDERS. Primary skin tumors can originate from epidermal cells, melanocytes, neuroendocrine (Merkel) cells, or dermal mesenchymal cells. In addition, metastatic tumors and hematopoietic or lymphoid malignancies (e.g., leukemia, lymphoma) can invade the skin.

A. Tumors of epidermal cells

1. Seborrheic keratosis ("senile wart") is a benign, exophytic outgrowth of the epidermal epithelium that is characterized by surface hyperkeratosis. Clinically, the lesions appear "stuck on" to the skin and can be removed easily by shave biopsy. Because the lesions may be pigmented, patients may be concerned about melanoma.

2. Actinic keratosis ("senile keratosis," "solar keratosis"), a lesion typically seen in older patients, is squamous cell carcinoma *in situ*. Lesions are typically seen on areas of the body that are prone to chronic sun exposure (e.g., the face, hands). Cytologic abnormalities are limited to the lower half of the epidermis.

3. Squamous cell carcinoma is an invasive cancer that has a tendency to metastasize. Lesions are often ulcerated with indurated margins; hyperkeratosis may be present.

4. Basal cell carcinoma, a locally invasive, low-grade malignancy, is the most common form of skin cancer. Small nodules, often ulcerated, are seen on areas of the skin that are exposed to sunlight.

B. Tumors of melanocytes. Pigmented lesions are common; most are benign but some are malignant.

1. Benign pigmented lesions
   a. Ephelides (freckles) are multiple pigmented macules that darken on exposure to sunlight and are typically seen in fair-skinned people.
   b. Lentigo (Latin, *"lentils"*) is discrete or solitary macular pigmentation that does not darken on exposure to sunlight.

2. Nevi
   a. Pigmented nevus (nevocellular nevus, "mole"). Pigmented nevi are benign congenital or acquired tumors of melanocytes.
   b. Dysplastic nevus is an atypical, irregular melanocytic lesion that is usually greater than 5 mm in diameter, with variegated pigmentation. Dysplastic nevi may be found on both sun-exposed and non–sun-exposed skin. When multiple and familial, dysplastic nevi may give rise to malignant melanoma (50% of cases) and must be regularly checked. Solitary and sporadic dysplastic nevi have a low malignant potential.

3. Malignant melanoma is a malignant tumor of melanocytes that occurs most often on sun-exposed parts of the body. Malignant melanoma may develop from nevi or normal skin and is classified as "superficial spreading," "nodular" or "acral lentiginous" (the latter form occurs in African-Americans as well as in whites).
   a. Clinical warning signs
      (1) Asymmetry
      (2) Border irregularity
      (3) Color variegation
      (4) Diameter greater than 6 mm
   b. Prognosis depends on the level of invasion of the dermis (Clark levels I–IV or Breslow measurements in millimeters).

17

Pathology of the Musculoskeletal System

I. DEVELOPMENTAL DISORDERS OF BONE

A. Achondroplasia is an autosomal dominant disorder. Mutation of the gene that encodes for the fibroblast growth factor receptor (FGFr) leads to disturbed endochondral ossification of the long bones.

   1. Heterozygous patients have short arms and legs. The trunk is normal and the head appears disproportionately large.

   2. Homozygous patients are severely deformed and die shortly after birth.

B. Osteogenesis imperfecta is a term used to refer to a group of diseases caused by mutations of the genes that encode for collagen type I.

   1. Four major forms of osteogenesis imperfecta are recognized, most of which are autosomal dominant disorders.

   2. The severity of the condition varies—some forms are lethal, whereas others cause only mild symptoms. Clinical findings include spontaneous fractures, joints that are easily dislocated, and blue sclerae.

C. Mucopolysaccharidoses are a group of seven disorders involving the accumulation of mucopolysaccharides (e.g., dermatan sulfate, keratan sulfate, chondroitin sulfate, heparan sulfate) in tissue. Patients have short limbs and stiff joints because normal mucopolysaccharides are essential for cartilage formation. In addition, patients often have mental retardation, coarse facial features, cardiac disease, and hepatosplenomegaly.

D. Osteopetrosis refers to a group of disorders characterized by failure of bone resorption as a result of osteoclast malfunction. These disorders may be either autosomal dominant or autosomal recessive. Clinical findings include thick, brittle bones and anemia and leukopenia (owing to the replacement of bone marrow by trabeculae).

II. METABOLIC DISORDERS OF BONE

A. Osteoporosis is loss of bone mass (osteopenia) characterized by the proportional loss of mineralized bone and nonmineralized osteoid. The trabeculae are thinner, with more space between them, predisposing the patient to fractures (Figure 17-1). Osteoporosis may be localized (e.g., found in a limb that has been immobilized or in the bone around an arthritic joint) or systemic.

   1. Causes of osteoporosis
      a. Primary osteoporosis exists in three forms—senile, postmenopausal, and id-

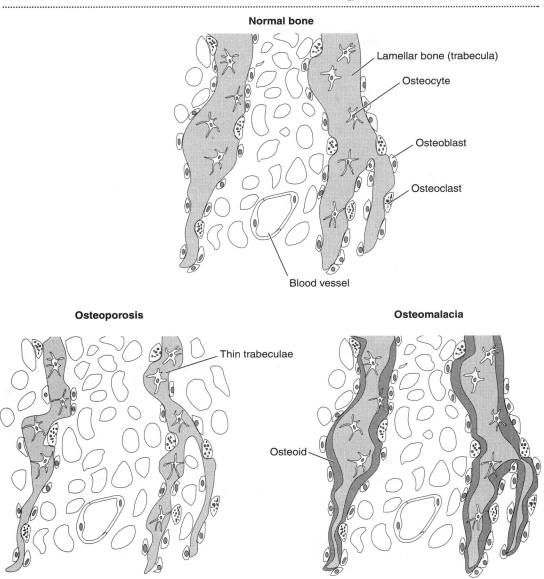

Figure 17-1.   In osteoporosis, the overall bone mass is decreased, but mineralization of the bone that remains is normal. This is in contrast to osteomalacia, which is characterized by defective mineralization.

iopathic of adulthood. The cause of primary osteoporosis is unknown, but certain factors predispose to the development of this condition:

(1) "Small-boned" frame
(2) Insufficient calcium and vitamin D intake
(3) Estrogen deficiency
(4) Sedentary lifestyle (weight bearing is important for bone remodeling!)

(5) Smoking
   b. Secondary osteoporosis. Causes are listed in Table 17-1.

2. Clinical diagnosis
   a. Signs and symptoms. In its early stages, osteoporosis is asymptomatic. Later, patients may present with compression fractures of the vertebrae, femoral head fractures, and slow healing of fractured bones.
   b. Imaging studies. Thinning of the cortex and trabeculae is best assessed using bone densitometry. Changes become apparent on radiographs only when more than 50% of the bone has been lost.

> **The blood calcium, potassium, parathyroid hormone (PTH), and vitamin D levels are normal in primary osteoporosis, in contrast to other osteopenias.**

3. Treatment. Primary osteoporosis is not treatable. In secondary osteoporosis, it is important to identify and treat the cause, if possible.

B. Osteomalacia and **rickets** are disorders characterized by softening of the bones as a result of vitamin D deficiency or abnormal vitamin D and phosphate metabolism. The trabeculae are "lined" with areas of nonmineralized osteoid (see Figure 17-1).

> **Osteomalacia occurs in bones that have already developed normally (i.e., in adults), whereas rickets occurs in the developing bones of children.**

1. Causes of osteomalacia and rickets include the following:
   a. Dietary deficiency of vitamin D
   b. Malabsorption syndromes
   c. Inadequate vitamin D synthesis (i.e., lack of sun exposure)
   d. Inadequate activation of vitamin D (i.e., kidney or liver disease)
   e. Inborn errors of vitamin D metabolism, such as those causing end-organ resistance ("vitamin D-resistant rickets")

2. Clinical diagnosis
   a. Signs and symptoms
      (1) Osteomalacia. Patients may complain of bone pain, but in adults, symptoms are rare.
      (2) Rickets. Children present with gross skeletal changes, such as bowing of the legs, enlargement of the costochondral junctions ("rachitic rosary"), and bosselation of the cranium ("rachitic tabes").

Table 17-1
Causes of Secondary Osteoporosis

Endocrine deficiency (e.g., adrenal, thyroid, or gonadal hormones)
Endocrine excess [e.g., parathyroid hormone (PTH), corticosteroids, growth hormone]
Nutritional deficiency (e.g., vitamin C or D deficiency, protein deficiency)
Pharmacologic therapy (e.g., lithium, anticoagulants, chemotherapeutic agents)
Neoplasia (e.g., hormonal paraneoplastic syndromes, bone metastases, multiple myeloma)

       b. **Imaging studies.** In osteomalacia, radiographs may show osteopenia. Bone deformities are typical of rickets.

C. **Hyperparathyroidism.** Excessive PTH levels cause activation of osteoclasts and osteoblasts, leading to bone loss, new bone formation, and ultimately, bone remodeling.

    1. **Pathologic findings** include:
       a. An increased number of osteoclasts within resorptive lacunae
       b. Osteoid that does not calcify
       c. Periarticular fibrosis

> **Owing to earlier diagnosis of hyperparathyroidism, severe bone lesions, such as bone cysts (osteitis fibrosa cystica) and brown tumors (i.e., large aggregates of osteoclasts) are rarely seen. Brown tumors are indistinguishable from giant cell tumors of bone.**

    2. **Laboratory findings** include increased serum PTH and calcium levels, and decreased serum phosphate levels.

D. **Renal osteodystrophy** is a term used to refer to the complex bone changes found in patients with end-stage kidney disease. Lesions are caused primarily by secondary hyperparathyroidism, lack of vitamin D activation, and metabolic acidosis associated with uremia.

    1. **Pathologic findings.** Bone lesions include a mixture of osteitis fibrosa cystica and osteomalacia. Metastatic calcifications are seen in various internal organs (e.g., lungs, stomach, kidneys).

    2. **Laboratory findings** include increased serum PTH, calcium, and phosphate levels.

E. **Paget disease** is a disease of unknown (possibly viral) etiology that is characterized by remodeling of bone and osteosclerosis ("mosaic-like" bone).

III. INFECTIOUS DISORDERS OF BONE

A. **Pyogenic osteomyelitis** is usually caused by *Staphylococcus aureus,* but may be caused by other bacteria, such as *Salmonella* species (e.g., in patients with sickle cell anemia). Infection may be acquired hematogenously, via direct inoculation (e.g., during an orthopedic procedure), or via extension from adjacent soft tissue, teeth, or joints.

    1. **Pathologic findings** include suppuration with localized liquefactive necrosis of the bone. The pus may drain from the bone to the skin through a sinus tract, or it may remain encapsulated (Brodie abscess).
       a. The **sequestrum** is detached necrotic bone within the abscess cavity.
       b. The **involucrum** is a rim of reactive new bone around the abscess.

> **Bone necrosis resulting from infection must be distinguished from aseptic (avascular) necrosis, which is much more common in the United States. Aseptic necrosis is caused by ischemia and most often involves the metaphysis of growing bones.**

    2. **Clinical findings** include systemic and local signs of infection, fractures, and bone deformities.

B. Tuberculous osteomyelitis, a complication of pulmonary tuberculosis, is rare in the United States. **Pott disease** (tuberculosis of the vertebrae) leads to a "hunchback" deformity.

C. Syphilitic osteomyelitis

1. **Congenital syphilis.** Skeletal abnormalities in children with syphilis include **periostitis, "saber shin"** (i.e., bent and thickened tibias), and **Hutchinson teeth** (i.e., deformed incisors). Radiographs of the skull reveal **"crewcut skull"** (i.e., hair-like spicules of new bone).

2. **Adult syphilis.** Gummas of the bone occur but are rare.

IV. NEOPLASTIC DISORDERS OF BONE

A. General considerations

1. **Sources of bone tumors**
   a. **Primary bone tumors.** The cells that give rise to primary bone tumors are summarized in Table 17-2.
   b. **Metastatic bone tumors.** Metastases to bone are more common than primary bone tumors.

2. **Age predilection.** Tumors appear in an age-dependent manner (Table 17-3).

3. **Anatomic distribution.** Each tumor type shows a preferential anatomic distribution (Figure 17-2).

4. **Metastatic tendencies.** Metastases typically spread hematogenously to the lungs.

B. Osteosarcoma. The neoplastic cells form osteoid or bone.

1. **Patients are usually between the ages of 10 and 20 years.** When osteosarcomas

Table 17-2
Histogenetic Classification of Primary Bone Tumors

Cells of Origin	Benign	Malignant
Bone cells	Osteoma	Osteosarcoma
	Osteoblastoma	
Cartilage cells	Chondroma	Chondrosarcoma
		Malignant fibrous histiocytoma
Osteoclasts	Giant cell tumor*	Giant cell tumor
Undifferentiated medullary cells	. . .	Ewing sarcoma
Plasma cells	. . .	Malignant myeloma
Fibroblasts	Fibroma	Malignant fibrous histiocytoma

*Although 90% of giant cell tumors are benign, 10% are malignant!

Table 17-3
Age Predilection for Primary Bone Tumors

Age of Patient	Type of Tumor
Younger than 19 years	Osteosarcoma, Ewing sarcoma
20–40 years	Giant cell tumors
40–60 years	Chondrosarcoma, multiple myeloma, malignant fibrous histiocytoma

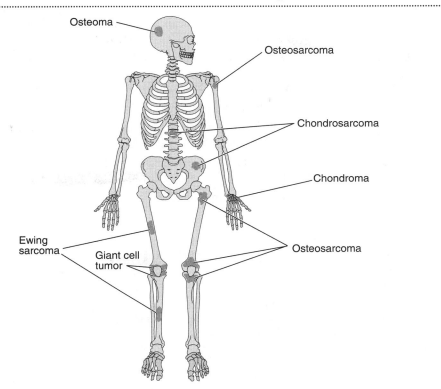

Figure 17-2. Anatomic predilection of primary bone tumors.

occur in elderly patients, they are often related to Paget disease and are associated with a poor prognosis.

2. Osteosarcomas show a predilection for the metaphyses of the long bones; 60% of tumors are located around the **knee.**

3. Tumor cells produce bone spicules, which account for radiographic signs such as the **"sunburst pattern"** and the **"Codman triangle"** sign (caused by elevation of the periosteum owing to subperiosteal new bone formation).

4. Treatment is based on **surgical resection,** which results in a 5-year survival rate of 60%.

> **Some forms of osteosarcoma (e.g., parosteal osteosarcoma) have a better prognosis than the conventional form.**

C. **Chondrosarcoma** is composed of malignant cartilage cells.

1. Patients are typically between the ages of 40 and 60 years.

2. The tumor shows a predilection for the **axial skeleton** (i.e., the pelvic and shoulder bones, vertebrae, and the proximal femur and humerus). Very rarely, chondrosarcomas occur in the small bones of the extremities.

3. Surgical resection results in a 5-year survival rate of 90% for grade I tumors, but only 40% for grade III tumors.

D. Ewing sarcoma is a member of the group of childhood tumors referred to as "small blue cell" tumors. Like the rest of these tumors, Ewing sarcoma is composed of sheets of primitive cells with small, round nuclei and glycogen-rich cytoplasm.

   1. Patients are typically between the ages of 5 and 20 years.

   2. The tumor has a predilection for the **diaphyses of the long bones.** It may occur in any bone and may be multifocal.

   3. The tumor cells extend from the medulla through the cortical bone and into the subperiosteal space, giving the bone an **"onion skin"** appearance on radiographs.

   4. Surgery combined with chemotherapy is associated with a 5-year survival rate of 60%.

V. JOINT DISORDERS

A. Degenerative joint disease (DJD, osteoarthritis) typically affects weight-bearing joints (e.g., the hip, knee, and intervertebral joints) and the interphalangeal joints.

   1. Causes
   a. Primary DJD is an **idiopathic age-related disease.** Mechanical stress on the joint cartilage and underlying bone is thought to play a role.
   b. Secondary DJD. Causes include:
      (1) Congenital deformities of the bones and joints (e.g., achondroplasia)
      (2) Metabolic disorders (e.g., the mucopolysaccharidoses)
      (3) Joint trauma
      (4) Neuropathic arthropathy (e.g., diabetic neuropathy)

   2. Pathologic findings (Figure 17-3). Thinning and fraying of the articular cartilage (fibrillation) is accompanied by destructive and reactive changes in the adjacent bone (e.g., eburnation, osteophyte formation, cyst formation).

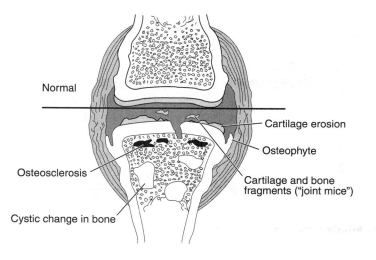

Figure 17-3. Pathologic findings in degenerative joint disease (DJD). Disruption of the ability of chondrocytes to maintain the articular cartilage leads to pathologic changes in the joint.

Heberden nodes and Bouchard nodes are osteophytes on the distal and proximal interphalangeal joints of the hands, respectively.

B. Rheumatoid arthritis is an autoimmune disorder that typically begins in the proximal interphalangeal and metacarpophalangeal joints of the hands and the small joints of the feet, and spreads to the wrist, elbow, ankle, and knee. The typical age at the time of onset is 30–60 years. Women are affected three times more often than men.

1. Pathologic findings
  a. **Articular pathology** (Figure 17-4). Changes are caused by inflammation of the synovium and include:
    (1) Chronic proliferative synovitis
    (2) Pannus ("cloak") formation over the articular cartilage
    (3) Cartilage erosion
    (4) Reactive osteoporosis in the adjacent bone
  b. **Extra-articular pathology**
    (1) **Skin.** Pathologic findings include subcutaneous nodules (less than 2 cm in diameter) showing fibrinoid necrosis surrounded by palisading histiocytes.
    (2) **Lungs.** Rheumatoid pneumoconiosis (Caplan syndrome) is rheumatoid arthritis in association with Coal Miners' Lung disease. Multiple, often confluent nodules are found throughout both lungs.

Felty syndrome is chronic rheumatoid arthritis in association with signs of hypersplenism (e.g., splenomegaly, neutropenia).

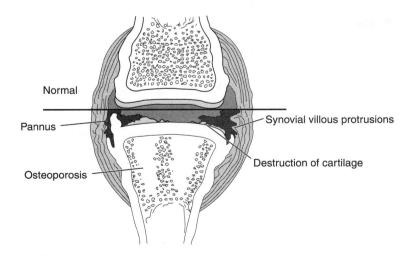

Normal

Pannus —

Osteoporosis —

— Synovial villous protrusions

— Destruction of cartilage

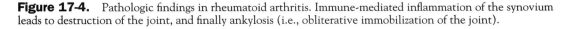

Figure 17-4.   Pathologic findings in rheumatoid arthritis. Immune-mediated inflammation of the synovium leads to destruction of the joint, and finally ankylosis (i.e., obliterative immobilization of the joint).

2. Laboratory findings. In most patients, rheumatoid factor (i.e., IgM antibodies against the Fc portion of IgG) can be detected in the serum.

3. Complications include joint deformity (e.g., "opera glass" deformities of the hands), joint stiffness, reduced mobility of the joint, and cardiopulmonary insufficiency.

C. Seronegative spondyloarthropathies. Features common to the seronegative spondyloarthropies include an association with **human leukocyte antigen-B27 (HLA-B27)** and an **absence of rheumatoid factor.**

1. Ankylosing spondylarthritis is a chronic progressive disease of unknown etiology that affects the small joints of the vertebral column and the sacroiliac joints. Men are affected nine times more often than women.

a. Patients experience progressive stiffening of the spine, beginning in early adulthood. On radiographs, ankylosis of the vertebral joints presents as **"bamboo-spine."** Eventually, the hips, shoulder, and knee joints are affected and may also become ankylotic.

b. HLA-B27 is present in 90% of patients.

2. Reiter syndrome is a disease of unknown etiology that most often affects young men and is characterized by the clinical triad of **arthritis, conjunctivitis,** and **sterile urethritis.** The arthritis usually involves the knee, ankle, and joints of the feet, but may spread to the spine.

 Reiter syndrome is often preceded by a gastrointestinal or genitourinary tract infection.

3. Psoriatic arthritis, which affects 5% of patients with psoriasis, is usually a mild disease. Spinal involvement is variable.

4. Enteropathic arthritis affects 10% of patients with ulcerative colitis or Crohn disease. Enteropathic arthritis is a migratory arthritis of the large joints and spine.

D. Gout is a disorder of purine metabolism characterized by hyperuricemia and the deposition of monosodium urate crystals in tissues, leading to arthritis and other disorders. Clinical manifestations include:

1. Podagra (i.e., pain in the metatarsophalangeal joint of the great toe)

2. Subcutaneous nodules (tophi) composed of monosodium urate)

3. Kidney disease (e.g., urolithiasis)

E. Infectious arthritis may be gonococcal (i.e., a complication of gonorrhea), streptococcal (i.e., a complication of systemic sepsis), spirochetal (i.e., a component of Lyme disease), or tuberculous.

VI. MUSCLE DISORDERS

A. Denervation atrophy may affect a single muscle fiber (e.g., as in diabetic neuropathy), a muscle fascicle [e.g., as in amyotrophic lateral sclerosis (ALS)], or an entire muscle or group of muscles (e.g., as in spinal cord trauma or transection).

B. Muscular dystrophies are a group of inherited disorders (Table 17-4) characterized by progressive degeneration and loss of muscle cells. Duchenne muscular dystrophy is the most common and most severe form of muscular dystrophy.

Table 17-4
Muscular Dystrophies

Type of Dystrophy	Inheritance	Incidence	Age at Onset (years)	Features
Duchenne	XR	1:3500	2–6	Progressive wasting of the pelvic and leg muscles eventually becomes generalized
Myotonic	AD	1:8000	20–30	Wasting of the facial and limb muscles with myotonia and typical electromyographic findings; extramuscular findings include baldness, gonadal atrophy, diabetes, cataracts, low IQ, and cardiomyopathy
Facioscapulohumeral	AD	1:20,000	10–20	Wasting of the facial and shoulder muscles; slow clinical progression
Becker	XR	1:35,000	10–30	Milder form of Duchenne dystrophy
Limb–girdle	AR	1:40,000	Variable	Wasting of the pelvic muscles progresses to the shoulder muscles; variable, usually mild to moderate, course

Modified with permission from Damjanov I, Conran PB, Goldblatt PJ: *Rypins' Intensive Reviews: Pathology.* Philadelphia, Lippincott-Raven, 1998, p 282.
AD = autosomal dominant; AR = autosomal recessive; IQ = intelligence quotient; XR = X-linked recessive.

C. **Inflammatory myopathies,** such as **polymyositis** and **dermatomyositis,** are immune-mediated disorders affecting primarily girls and young women.

When inflammatory myopathies occur in older patients, they are usually part of a paraneoplastic syndrome.

D. **Myasthenia gravis** is an autoimmune muscle disease characterized by periodic episodes of weakness caused by binding of antibodies to acetylcholine (ACh) receptors at the neuromuscular junction. The extraocular muscles, facial muscles, and muscles of mastication are most often involved; in advanced cases, the diaphragm is involved as well.

E. **Neoplastic disorders of skeletal muscle** include **rhabdomyosarcoma,** a tumor of childhood.

18

Pathology of the Nervous System

I. DEVELOPMENTAL DISORDERS

A. **Dysraphic disorders (neural tube defects)** are multifactorial in origin.

1. **Anencephaly** (i.e., lack of the cerebral hemispheres and calvaria) is incompatible with life.

2. **Spinal neural tube defects.** Defects range in severity (Figure 18-1).

B. **Inborn errors of metabolism**

1. **Lysosomal storage diseases**
   a. **Gangliosidoses. Tay-Sachs disease** is caused by **α-hexosaminidase deficiency,** which leads to the accumulation of gangliosides in the neurons and glial cells throughout the central and peripheral nervous systems.
   b. **Mucopolysaccharidoses** (see Chapter 17 I C). The accumulation of mucopolysaccharides in neurons accounts for the mental retardation that is often a component of these disorders.

2. **Leukodystrophies.** In these conditions, a metabolic abnormality interferes with the body's ability to produce or maintain myelin. The most common leukodystrophies are:
   a. **Metachromatic leukodystrophy** (arylsulfatase A deficiency)
   b. **Krabbe disease** (β-galactosidase deficiency)
   c. **Adrenoleukodystrophy** (peroxisomal defect)

C. **Phakomatoses (hereditary neurocutaneous syndromes)**

1. **Neurofibromatosis**
   a. **Type I** is characterized by multiple neurofibromas, meningiomas, and café-au-lait spots.
   b. **Type II** is characterized by vestibulocochlear nerve schwannomas and meningiomas.

2. **Tuberous sclerosis** is characterized by hamartomas of the cerebral cortex (tubers), retina, and viscera in association with skin lesions (e.g., subungual fibromas; and facial angiofibromas).

3. **von Hippel-Lindau disease** is characterized by hemangioblastomas of the cerebellum and retina and renal, hepatic, and pancreatic cysts.

II. CIRCULATORY DISORDERS

A. **Cerebral infarcts** have four major causes:

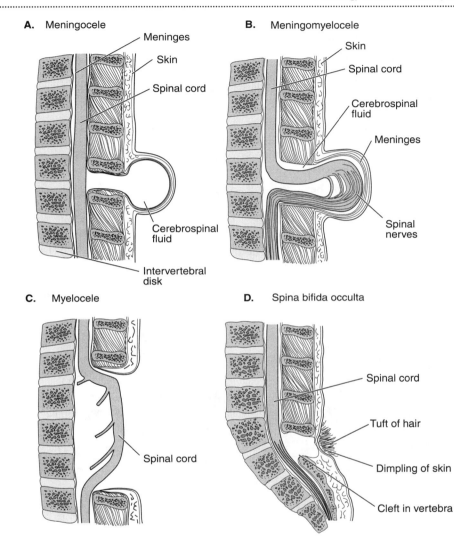

A. Meningocele

Meninges
Skin
Spinal cord
Cerebrospinal fluid
Intervertebral disk

B. Meningomyelocele

Skin
Spinal cord
Cerebrospinal fluid
Meninges
Spinal nerves

C. Myelocele

Spinal cord

D. Spina bifida occulta

Spinal cord
Tuft of hair
Dimpling of skin
Cleft in vertebra

Figure 18-1. Spinal neural tube defects. (A) Meningocele is herniation of the meninges, unaccompanied by the spinal cord. (B) Meningomyelocele is herniation of the meninges and spinal cord. (C) Myelocele is herniation of the spinal cord, without any protective covering. (D) Spina bifida occulta. There is a defect in the neural tube, but the skin is intact and the meninges and spinal cord are not herniated. Externally, the defect may be marked by a dimple in the skin or a tuft of hair.

1. **Thrombosis** of the cerebral arteries is usually a complication of atherosclerosis.

2. **Embolism.** The middle cerebral artery is most prone to occlusion by an embolus.

3. **Hypotension.** Hypotensive infarcts usually involve the "watershed" areas (i.e., areas where the peripheral arteries of two vascular beds meet) and the deep layers of the cortex.

4. **Hypertension.** Lacunae (i.e., multiple cystic infarcts, most prominent in the basal

ganglia) are caused by arteriolar occlusion in patients with hypertensive cere-brovascular disease.

B. Intracranial hemorrhages (Figure 18-2)

1. **Epidural hematoma** is caused by acute traumatic rupture of the middle meningeal artery (e.g., following a skull fracture). The middle meningeal artery is contained within the epidural space.

2. **Subdural hematoma** is caused by disruption of the bridging veins, which extend between the brain and the dural sinuses. Subdural hematomas contain clotted blood and are usually caused by repetitive trauma (e.g., boxing injuries, "shaken baby" syndrome).

3. **Subarachnoid hemorrhage** is an acute massive hemorrhage caused by rupture of a berry aneurysm (i.e., a saccular aneurysm typically arising from the circle of Willis at the base of the brain).

4. **Intracerebral hemorrhage** has many causes:

   a. **Trauma.** Shearing of the intraparenchymal vessels can lead to intracerebral hemorrhage. Shear injuries are caused by rapid acceleration or deceleration, such as would occur in a motor vehicle collision).

   b. **Uncontrolled hypertension** can lead to rupture of an intraparenchymal ves-

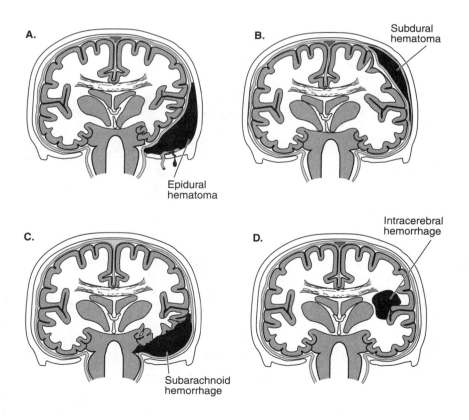

Figure 18-2. Intracranial hemorrhages.

sel. Hemorrhages of this type usually occur in the basal ganglia (70% of cases), cerebellum (20% of cases), and pons (10% of cases).

   c. **Infarction.** Hemorrhage into an infarct may occur, especially when the infarct involves arterial "watershed" areas or was caused by transient occlusion of the artery (e.g., by an embolus that is subsequently lysed).

III. INFECTIOUS DISORDERS. Routes of infection include **direct inoculation** (e.g., following penetrating trauma), **hematogenous spread** (e.g., as a complication of sepsis, pneumonia, or pharyngitis), **local extension** (e.g., from the nasal sinuses or mastoid bone), and **retrograde axonal migration** (e.g., as in rabies).

A. Meningitis

   1. **Acute meningitis.** Pathologic findings include inflammation of the meninges accompanied by an exudate of polymorphonuclear neutrophils (PMNs) or lymphocytes in the subarachnoid space.

     a. **Bacterial meningitis** is most often caused by *Escherichia coli* (in neonates), *Haemophilus influenzae* (in infants and children), and *Neisseria meningitidis* or *Streptococcus pneumoniae* (in adults).

     b. **Viral meningitis.** The most common viral causes of acute meningitis are **coxsackievirus** and **echovirus.**

   2. **Chronic meningitis.** In chronic meningitis, the subarachnoid space contains infiltrates of lymphocytes, plasma cells, macrophages, or granulomas.

     a. **Tuberculous meningitis.** The meninges on the basal aspect of the brain are most often affected.

     b. **Syphilitic meningitis.** Patients with tertiary syphilis may present with signs of meningitis (so-called meningovascular syphilis).

     c. **Cryptococcal meningitis** is common in patients with AIDS.

> **Other opportunistic fungi that can cause chronic meningitis include *Candida albicans*, *Aspergillus* species, and *Mucor* species.**

B. **Encephalitis** is generalized infection of the brain parenchyma, most often caused by viruses. Intracerebral infection is followed by brain cell necrosis. The accompanying lymphocytic infiltrate is most prominent around the blood vessels. Causes include the following:

   1. **Arthropod-borne viruses** (e.g., **Eastern equine encephalitis virus, Western equine encephalitis virus, St. Louis encephalitis virus**) are associated with epidemic diffuse encephalitides.

   2. **Herpesviruses**

     a. **Herpes simplex virus-1 (HSV-1)** causes a necrotizing hemorrhagic encephalitis of the inferior temporal lobe, most often in children and young adults.

     b. **Herpes simplex virus-2 (HSV-2)** causes a generalized encephalitis in 50% of infants born to women with primary genital HSV-2 infection.

   3. **Rabies virus.** Negri bodies, neuronal necrosis, and lymphocytic infiltrates are most prominent in the neurons of the hippocampus and in the Purkinje cells of the cerebellum.

   4. **JC polyoma virus** invades the oligodendroglia, resulting in demyelination [progressive multifocal leukoencephalopathy (PML)]. PML is most common in immunocompromised patients.

5. Measles virus. Subacute sclerosing panencephalitis is a rare complication that develops several years after primary measles virus infection. Pathologic findings include intranuclear inclusion bodies in the oligodendroglia, areas of demyelination and gliosis, and inflammation.

6. HIV. HIV encephalitis, a feature of AIDS, is clinically associated with progressive dementia and motor disturbances. Pathologic findings include microglial nodules with multinucleated giant cells.

C. Prion diseases. Altered prion protein (PrP) causes spongiform encephalopathies.

1. Creutzfeldt-Jakob disease is characterized by progressive dementia and death within 6–7 months. Most cases are sporadic, but some are familial.

2. Kuru is a progressive, fatal neurologic disease affecting members of a tribe in New Guinea. Kuru is associated with a form of ritualistic cannibalism that involves eating the brains of deceased members of the tribe.

3. Gerstmann-Sträussler disease is a hereditary form of slowly progressive dementia.

IV. IMMUNE-MEDIATED DISORDERS include **multiple sclerosis,** a disease characterized by the episodic appearance of neurologic deficits beginning during the third decade. Initially, the deficits regress, but they eventually recur and become progressively more severe.

A. Cause. It is thought that both environmental and familial factors contribute to the development of the autoimmunity against myelin components that is seen in multiple sclerosis.

1. The concordance rate is 25% in identical twins.

2. Multiple sclerosis is more common in cold climates.

B. Pathologic findings. Areas of demyelination (i.e, **plaques)** are commonly seen around the ventricles, in the medulla and cerebellum, on the optic nerve, and in the spinal cord.

1. Acute lesions are usually soft, pale pink, and accompanied by a lymphocytic infiltrate. A few axonal processes may be noted. In active lesions, demyelination is evidenced by the presence of macrophages containing lipids.

2. Old lesions. Inactive plaques, which may be gray, are composed of demyelinated axons with some gliosis but no inflammatory cells.

C. Clinical findings. The course is unpredictable: 75% of patients survive for as long as 25 years, but 10% experience a rapid decline.

1. History and physical examination. Signs and symptoms, which usually last 2–4 months, resolve, and then return in about 2 years. Depending on the location of the lesion, signs and symptoms may include:
   a. Visual problems (e.g., blurring, loss of the visual field, diplopia)
   b. Paresthesia
   c. Motor disturbances affecting gait
   d. Speech disorders

2. Laboratory studies. Oligoclonal immunoglobulins are detected in the cerebrospinal fluid (CSF).

3. **Imaging studies.** Periventricular plaques are visible on head computed tomography (CT) scans.

V. TOXIC OR METABOLIC DISORDERS

A. **Wernicke encephalopathy** is caused by **vitamin B$_1$ (thiamine) deficiency,** a deficiency most often seen in the settings of alcoholism or chronic gastric disease.

    1. **Pathologic findings** include hemorrhage and small vessel proliferation in the mammillary bodies of the hypothalamus, parts of the thalamus, the pons, and the medulla oblongata.

    2. **Clinical findings** include confusion of sudden onset, paralysis of the extraocular muscles, ataxia, and irreversible memory loss **(Korsakoff psychosis).**

B. **Subacute combined degeneration** is caused by **vitamin B$_{12}$ (cobalamin) deficiency,** a deficiency most often seen in the setting of type A gastritis (see Chapter 10 II D 2 a).

    1. **Pathologic findings** include myelin vacuolation and degeneration in the dorsal and lateral white matter of the spinal cord.

    2. **Clinical findings** include an abnormal gait (owing to loss of proprioception and ataxia), spastic weakness of the legs that may progress to paraplegia, and confusion ("psychosis," "megaloblastic madness").

> Remember the **five Ps** of vitamin B$_{12}$ deficiency:
> **Parietal cell loss in the stomach (type A gastritis)**
> **Pernicious anemia**
> **Proprioceptor loss (loss of position and vibration sense)**
> **Paresthesias**
> **Psychosis ("megaloblastic madness")**

VI. NEURODEGENERATIVE DISORDERS

A. **Alzheimer disease** is the most common form of dementia (i.e., loss of all cognitive function) in the United States. The incidence increases with age—while only 1% of 60-year-old men and women have Alzheimer disease, 40% of those who are 85 years or older have this type of dementia. Women are affected three times more often than men.

    1. **Causes.** Most cases are sporadic (90%). However, the occurrence of some familial cases suggests that genetic risk factors exist for the disease:
        a. A specific allele of apolipoprotein E, is found in familial cases
        b. Genes for familial Alzheimer disease and the β-amyloid precursor protein, are both on chromosome 21
        c. Mutated genes for presenilins I and II, are found in familial cases

    2. **Pathologic findings** (Figure 18-3)
        a. **Gross findings** can be observed on a CT scan or at autopsy and include:
            (1) **Cortical atrophy** (narrow gyri, wide sulci)
            (2) **Dilated lateral ventricles** (hydrocephalus *ex vacuo*)
        b. **Microscopic findings** include:
            (1) **Neuritic (senile) plaques** with a central core composed of β-amyloid
            (2) **Neurofibrillary tangles**

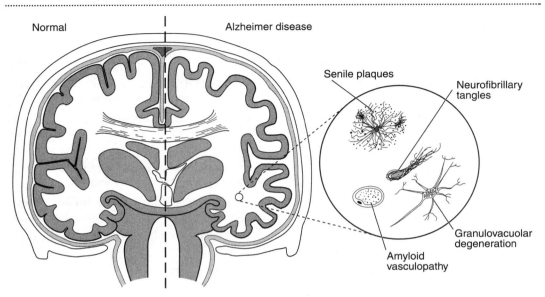

Figure 18-3. Gross and microscopic pathologic changes in Alzheimer disease. Generalized loss of the brain parenchyma results in atrophied gyri and widened sulci. Loss and degeneration of neurons is evidenced by neuritic (senile) plaques, neurofibrillary tangles, and granulovacuolar degeneration. In addition to forming the core of the neuritic plaques, β-amyloid is deposited in the walls of the small blood vessels of the brain.

> **(3)** Granulovacuolar degeneration
> **(4)** Amyloid angiopathy

  3. Clinical findings. There is a progressive deterioration from subtle to severe dementia. Patients experience loss of short-term memory, disorientation in time and space, and difficulty with language (i.e., understanding and expressing words).

B. Parkinsonism is a syndrome characterized by rigidity, tremor, an expressionless facies, a stooped posture, and a festinating gait (i.e., involuntary small, fast steps).

  1. Causes. Parkinsonism may be **idiopathic** (in which case it is referred to as Parkinson disease or paralysis agitans), or secondary (i.e., **induced by drugs, trauma, encephalitis,** or other insults).

  2. Pathologic findings. Lesions involve the clusters of pigmented nerve cells in the brain stem (i.e., the substantia nigra and the locus ceruleus).

   a. In parkinsonism, the substantia nigra and locus ceruleus are pale, owing to **loss of neuromelanin-containing neurons.**

   b. The remaining neurons contain eosinophilic cytoplasmic inclusions composed of synuclein-1 **(Lewy bodies).**

  3. Clinical findings. The disease progressively worsens, often leading to complete immobility within 10–15 years. Many patients die as a result of intercurrent infections brought about by limited mobility, or as a result of trauma sustained during falls (which become more frequent as postural instability worsens).

C. Huntington disease is an autosomal dominant disease characterized by chorea and progressive dementia. The onset of symptoms typically does not occur until the fourth decade.

1. Pathogenesis. Mutation of the Huntington gene, located on chromosome 4, results in an increased number of trinucleotide repeats and the production of mutant huntingtin. The mutant huntingtin is thought to negatively affect a protein that is responsible for normal functioning of the extrapyramidal motor system. Gliosis and loss of the small neurons in the basal ganglia accounts for the extrapyramidal symptoms (e.g., chorea), while loss of neurons in the cortex causes the dementia.

> **Because the disorder is thought to result from aberrant function of the mutant huntingtin (as opposed to loss of function of normal huntingtin), the mutation responsible for Huntington disease is referred to as a "gain of function" mutation.**

2. Pathologic findings include atrophy of the caudate nucleus, putamen and globus pallidus, symmetric ("box-like") dilatation of the lateral ventricles, and loss of neurons in the basal ganglia and cortex.

3. Clinical findings include choreoathetotic involuntary movements (with or without rigidity), depression and suicidal behavior, and dementia. The patient's clinical condition progressively deteriorates over the course of 10–20 years.

D. Amyotrophic lateral sclerosis (ALS) is a progressive degenerative disease involving the lower and upper motor neurons of the pyramidal system.

1. Cause. Most cases are sporadic, but 10% are autosomal dominant, and some are related to mutation of the gene for superoxide dismutase.

2. Pathologic findings include:
   a. Loss of motor neurons in the anterior horn, brain stem, and cortex
   b. Loss of corticospinal fibers in the lateral and anterior columns of the spinal cord
   c. Atrophy of the peripheral nerves owing to loss of the motor axons
   d. Denervation atrophy of the skeletal muscles

3. Clinical findings. Patients loose muscle strength but live for an average of 5 years before succumbing to respiratory insufficiency. Early in the disease course, spasticity and hyperactive deep tendon reflexes are seen.

VII. NEOPLASTIC DISORDERS OF THE CENTRAL NERVOUS SYSTEM (CNS)

A. General considerations

1. Origin of brain tumors
   a. Primary brain tumors (Table 18-1)
   b. Metastatic brain tumors. The ratio of primary to metastatic tumors in the brain is 50:50. Most often, metastatic brain tumors occur secondary to lung cancer, breast cancer, colorectal cancer, renal carcinoma, or malignant melanoma.

Table 18-1
Incidence and Origin of Primary Brain Tumors

Tumor Type	Incidence	Cell of Origin
Glioblastoma multiforme	40%	Astrocytes
Astrocytoma	20%	Astrocytes
Meningioma	15%	Meningothelial cells
Medulloblastoma	10%	Neural cell precursors*
Schwannoma	8%	Schwann cells
Oligodendroglioma	3%	Oligodendroglial cells
Ependymoma	3%	Ependymal cells

*Adult neurons are postmitotic cells and do not give rise to tumors!

To remember the sources of metastases to the brain, use the mnemonic "BREAST:"
Breast
Renal
Enteric
Airway and
Skin (especially melanoma)
Tumors of any origin can metastasize to the brain!

2. **Age predilection.** Most brain tumors occur during adulthood, with the exception of medulloblastoma, pilocytic astrocytoma, and most ependymomas, which occur in children.

3. **Anatomic distribution.** Each tumor type shows a preferential anatomic distribution (Figure 18-4).

4. **Metastatic tendencies.** Generally speaking, brain tumors do not metastasize!

B. Gliomas

1. **Glioblastoma multiforme,** the **most common type of primary brain tumor,** is invariably lethal within 8–12 months.
   a. **Tumor features.** Glioblastoma multiforme most often arises in patients between the ages of 40 and 60 years, usually in the cerebral hemispheres. The tumor exhibits infiltrative growth and may be bilateral.
   b. **Pathologic findings.** The name "multiforme" is derived from the tumor's variegated gross and microscopic appearance.

2. **Astrocytoma** accounts for 20% of all primary brain tumors, and is the second most common tumor of the spinal cord (after ependymoma). Cystic astrocytomas occur in the cerebellum, in children. Most patients die within 5–7 years.

3. **Oligodendroglioma,** a slow-growing, circumscribed (i.e., low-grade) malignant tumor, is the glioma with the best overall prognosis (patients usually survive for at least 10 years). Oligodendroglioma arises in the cerebral hemispheres of patients between the ages of 30 and 50 years.

C. **Ependymoma** is a slow-growing malignant tumor of the ependymal cells, which line

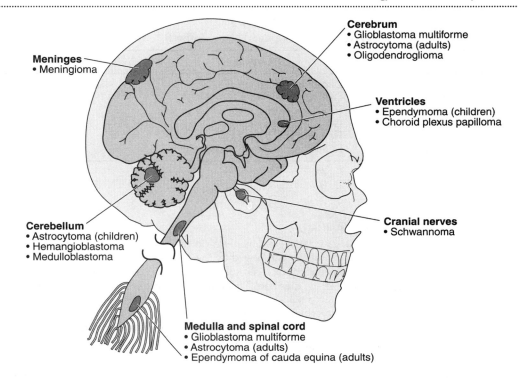

Figure 18-4. Anatomic predilection of primary brain tumors. All brain tumors are malignant, except for meningioma and schwannoma.

the choroid plexus and ventricles and secrete CSF. In children, these tumors most often arise in the fourth ventricle, whereas in adults, they are most commonly located in the spinal cord and cauda equina.

D. **Medulloblastoma,** a malignant cerebellar tumor of undifferentiated neural cell precursors, accounts for 60% of childhood primary central nervous system (CNS) tumors (but only 10% of primary CNS tumors overall). Treatment with radiation and chemotherapy is associated with a 5-year survival rate of 75%; however, if left untreated, the tumor is lethal within 1–2 years.

E. **Meningiomas** are benign tumors that arise from the meningothelial cells of the arachnoid mater. They may compress the brain or permeate the overlying bone. In most cases, the prognosis is excellent.

F. **Schwannoma** is a benign tumor that originates from the Schwann cells of cranial nerve VIII and is located in the cerebellopontine angle.

VIII. DISORDERS OF THE PERIPHERAL NERVOUS SYSTEM

A. **Peripheral neuropathy** is a general term used to describe loss of normal sensory or motor peripheral nerve function.

1. **Causes.** Peripheral neuropathy has many causes (Table 18-2).

Table 18-2
Causes of Peripheral Neuropathy

Category	Example
Mechanical disorders	Carpal tunnel syndrome, trauma
Metabolic disorders	Diabetes*, amyloidosis
Toxic disorders	Heavy metals
Immune-mediated disorders	Guillain-Barré syndrome
Infectious disorders	Herpes zoster, leprosy
Congenital disorders	Charcot-Marie-Tooth disease

*The most common cause.

2. General patterns of injury

   a. **Wallerian degeneration** is degeneration of the axons distal to a site of transection. Degeneration is followed by regeneration.

   b. **Primary axonal degeneration** results from injury to the neuron associated with the axon; the axon "dies back" from its distal end. Many forms of injury (e.g., toxic or ischemic insults) result in primary axonal degeneration.

   c. **Segmental demyelination** of peripheral nerves (i.e., loss of the myelin sheath) is often a component of immune-mediated or infectious neuropathy.

B. **Peripheral nerve tumors** include **neurofibroma** and **schwannoma,** both of which are benign, and **malignant peripheral nerve sheath tumors,** which are rare. Multiple peripheral nerve tumors (of all three types) may be seen in patients with neurofibromatosis type I.

Index

References in *italics* indicate figures; those followed by "t" denote tables